Weight
Understanding ... ... Fat

Weight Loss
for
Health Gain

Understanding the Metabolism of Fat

Dr Joe Fitzgibbon

Newleaf

Newleaf
an imprint of
Gill & Macmillan Ltd
Hume Avenue, Park West
Dublin 12
with associated companies throughout the world
www.gillmacmillan.ie

© Dr Joe Fitzgibbon 2003
0 7171 3568 3

Index compiled by Cover To Cover
Design by Anú Design
Print origination by Redbarn Publishing
Printed by the Woodprintcraft Group Ltd, Dublin

This book is typeset in AdobeGaramond 10 on 15 point

The paper used in this book is made from the wood pulp of managed forests. For every tree felled, at least one tree is planted, thereby renewing natural resources.

A CIP catalogue record for this book is available from the British Library.

1 3 5 4 2

Contents

Glossary

adipose tissue: cells which store fat
adrenaline: the hormone responsible for the 'flight or fight' response

blood pressure: the amount of work the heart has to exert to pump blood through the arteries
BMI: Body Mass Index; a measure of body weight in relation to height
BMR: Basal Metabolic Rate; the minimum energy required by the body at rest

calorie: a unit of energy; the amount of heat required to raise the temperature of 1 gram of water by 1°C
carbohydrate: a compound of carbon, hydrogen and oxygen commonly known as sugars, starches or non-starch polysaccharides
cholesterol: a fatty steroid alcohol which may cause arteriosclerosis if present in excess
chronic: long-lasting

diabetes mellitus: a disease characterised by excessive thirst, excessive hunger and passing excessive urine
digestion: the ingestion, break-down and absorption of food
disaccharide: two single sugar units bound together

embolism: a clot that travels through blood vessels until it can no longer fit through; it then lodges and obstructs blood flow
energy: the ability to do work
enzyme: any protein that catalyses (speeds up) a biochemical reaction

fat/s: triacylglycerols; three fatty acids linked to a glycerol unit
food intolerance: any abnormal response to food that causes symptoms

glucose: the most common single sugar unit
glycogen: a series of glucose units linked together

HDL-cholesterol: a high-density lipoprotein attached to cholesterol, making it a 'good form of cholesterol'

heart attack: a serious event in which part of the heart muscle is deprived of blood supply

hormone: a substance produced by one part of the body which travels to and affects other parts of the body

hypertension: high blood pressure

hypothalamus: a part of the brain that regulates hormone secretion

insulin: the hormone secreted by the pancreas which (a) promotes the entry of glucose into cells, (b) promotes the synthesis of protein, and (c) inhibits the breakdown of fat

joule: a unit of energy; 1 joule = 0.239 calories

kilocalorie (kcal): a unit of energy; 1 kcal = 1,000 calories

kilojoule: 1,000 joules

LDL-cholesterol: a low-density lipoprotein attached to cholesterol, making it a 'bad form of cholesterol'

lipoprotein: a protein linked to a lipid by a bond

macronutrient: proteins, carbohydrates and fats are referred to as macronutrients

metabolism: the sum of biochemical reactions in the body

monosaccharide: a single sugar unit

morbid/morbidity: causing or relating to illness

obesity: excessive body fat, defined as a BMI greater than 30

PAL: Physical Activity Level; an estimate of how much physical activity takes place during various activities and occupations

pancreas: an organ that produces enzymes for digestion, and hormones that control blood sugar

physiology: the function of organs in the body

polysaccharide: more than two single sugar units bound together

protein: a series of amino acids linked together by bonds

satiation: the process of reaching satiety

satiety: the feeling of fullness after meals which inhibits further food intake

stroke: a serious event in which part of the brain is deprived of blood supply

thrombosis: blood clot

thyroid: a gland in the neck that produces the hormone thyroxine

thyroxine: hormone from the thyroid gland that regulates the metabolism of the whole body

toxic: poisonous

triglyceride: see fat/s

Introduction

As a society, we spend a fortune each year on what has become known as the 'slimming industry'. We splash out on every new product that promises to make us look slimmer and fitter, and especially if it claims to do so quickly and easily. We buy pills and potions and various other aids in our quest for weight loss. By and large, they don't work.

We are targeted by advertising campaigns to buy low-fat, low-calorie foods and 'diet' drinks. The industry is cashing in on our competing desires for good-tasting food and slim bodies. They reinforce their message by both subliminal and overt images, in which slimness is equated with attractiveness, energy and happiness. Some companies are even trying to invent zero-calorie foods that will taste as good as the real thing – non-fattening ice cream and chocolate, for instance. They, too, are trying to exploit our dilemma.

Countless articles and books have been written on the subject of diet and weight loss. Many of these claim to have found 'the answer', a hitherto undiscovered dietary mystery hidden for generations from mere mortals like you and me! These often give conflicting advice: cut out the sugar, stop eating starch, stay away from bread, avoid yeast, and so on. Some of these can only be described as fad diets, having no basis whatsoever in science. The one thing they all have in common is this:

the promise of a quick and easy path to the body shape you've always dreamt of. But far from solving our problem, such gimmicks only add to our confusion, and then to our despair when we eventually admit defeat. And there is plenty of defeat: 95 per cent of people who successfully lose weight put it back on again within a few short years.

At the present time, our society emulates and rewards thinness, and places enormous emphasis on appearance. We are encouraged to buy the product and lose weight in order to *look* good. These attitudes have several detrimental effects. Our teenage girls are driven to distraction with unrealistic expectations of so-called beauty; the overweight amongst us are scorned, and the obese suffer discrimination. Perhaps this is why almost a half of all non-pregnant women are currently trying to lose excess weight, and a further third are consciously trying to avoid putting it on.

Health promotion agencies emphasise the health aspects of diet and body weight. They tell us that we can add length and health to our days by choosing the right foods. Sadly, and in spite of several sustained educational campaigns, they too have failed to change the basic facts: some 40–50 per cent of adults in Western societies are overweight, and up to 20 per cent are obese – figures which are rising with each passing year. This trend is also evident in some of the former socialist economies. These rates led the World Health Organisation to declare, in 1997, that obesity has become a global epidemic – an epidemic that looks certain to continue because our children, as they so often do, are following in our footsteps. At the present rate of increase the entire population of Western societies could be overweight or obese by the end of this century. Overweight and obesity, and their adverse effects on health, are set to become the single most important public health issue of our time. Indeed, obesity is overtaking smoking as the single most important cause of avoidable ill-health.

Some fortunate people will never get fat. They can eat to their hearts' content and yet never seem to worry about their body weight.

The rest of us will need to be more careful. Two-thirds of all overweight adults gained the excess weight during their adult years. The other third were overweight as children and simply stayed overweight, or became even more overweight through their adult years. Thus, you may say of yourself that you 'have always been a little on the plump side', or even that you have 'always been big'. On the other hand, you may have started out quite slim and trim, but slowly and imperceptibly gained weight with each passing year. Do you now have to peer over your abdomen to see the dial on the weighing scales? Are your clothes feeling tight? And, if so, have you tried to convince yourself that they shrank in the wash? Perhaps you squeezed into them anyway, but have you been squeezed into submission? Have you bought the next size up? And the next? Well, that's the way it happens for most of us. A slow but relentless spread.

Overweight and obesity pose a serious threat to health. This is why doctors and other health professionals tend to go on and on about the importance of losing excess weight and maintaining ideal weight. But as every overweight person knows, it is much easier to talk about losing weight than to actually achieve it. Countless genuine overweight and obese people have tried and failed to lose weight; and they have done so time and time again. Many of these are now left with the awful impression that they simply cannot lose weight. But they can.

This book explains, in simple terms, the process of weight gain and the effects of weight on health. It also offers simple and pragmatic advice on what you can do about it. You *can* lose weight. You *can* add length and health to your days. And you can do all of that without starving yourself to death!

Section 1

Understanding Fat

1

Fat – The Bigger Picture

This book is written for those who are concerned about body weight. Generally speaking, there are two principal sources of concern which most of us share. The first relates to the various psycho-social issues surrounding fatness and body image; the second relates to the health consequences of being overweight or obese. Both of these are important.

Body image is a fundamental part of how we see ourselves in general. This is something we all know by intuition, but the truth of it was brought home to me as a young doctor in postgraduate training. The consultant and I were chatting at the end of another busy morning in the psychiatric out-patients' clinic. He pointed out the rarity of finding someone who is fully happy with his or her body. 'Most of us would change our body shape', he announced, 'in one way or another, if we were given the opportunity. We would rather be taller or shorter; or have smaller feet, more muscles, fewer spots, no blemishes, bigger breasts, smaller breasts, a more rounded nose, straighter teeth, more weight or a thinner waist!' He reminded me that the popular appeal of cosmetic surgery merely reflects this common discontent. Then he wrapped up his impromptu lesson: 'Individuals who are entirely happy with their body image tend to be very psychologically stable.' He was not referring to those who put great effort into their physical appearance; nor to those who through the good fortunes of genetic inheritance are well proportioned and naturally good looking. He was referring to the innate contentment which accompanies self-acceptance – warts and all. It is indeed a great gift to be able to accept ourselves as we are, complete with our physical individuality, whether we be thin, fat or anywhere in between.

Many obese persons will readily admit that they suffer some degree of psychological impact as a direct result of their 'weight problem'. They frequently feel bad about themselves, their fat and their appearance. For some, their self-esteem may be severely challenged. Others put on a brave and jolly face, and would seem to endorse the notion we inherit from folklore; namely, that fat people are thick-skinned, larger than life, and live life to the full. But the sad fact is that overweight and obesity are associated with quite the opposite characteristics: depression and poor self-image. All of this is compounded by the pervasively rude and moralistic attitudes which are meted out to the overweight by those who, for some strange reason, consider themselves entitled to pass judgement. Tacit accusations ranging from gluttony to slovenliness are frequently invoked and poorly disguised. The truth is that these vices have little if anything to do with the vast majority of ordinary people who happen to be overweight. Nevertheless, the overweight are teased and bullied, and may even find themselves at the receiving end of downright hostility and discrimination.

Social attitudes are fickle and subject to change. There was a time when 'plumpness' was considered attractive, and when our present-day skin-and-bone supermodels would have been shunned in favour of those with a little more fat. Social attitudes are also subject to cultural influence. For example, obesity is treasured in some societies as a status symbol: 'Look at me! I'm fat because I can afford good food and my servants do all the hard work.' Likewise, some cultures would question a husband whose wife does not fatten during their first year of marriage: her failure to gain weight would lead in-laws to suspect that their daughter was not being properly cared for! It seems clear, then, that the psychological burden of the overweight is determined by the dominant attitudes of the society in which we live.

This book will focus particularly on the health aspects of weight. Since I am neither a psychologist nor a sociologist, I am not qualified to delve into the important issues of psychology and sociology. However, I believe that a full understanding of the health aspects of weight will lead us away from futile and harmful anxieties over appearance, into a much more positive frame of mind.

THE MOST COMPELLING REASON FOR LOSING WEIGHT

The Metropolitan Life Assurance Company issued a report in 1937 which drew attention to the importance of body weight in relation to life expectancy. They were amongst the first to prove that being overweight was a significant risk factor for premature death. Needless to say, their interest in all of this was not medical, but financial – they wanted to reduce their exposure to early payouts. Having now demonstrated conclusively that the overweight were much more likely to die young and have their policies cashed in, the company felt justified in charging them higher premiums for life cover in the first place. The association between excess body weight and mortality was independent of all other known risk factors such as cigarette smoking, high blood pressure, family history, and so forth. These early findings have been confirmed by subsequent large-scale studies and are now widely accepted by health professionals internationally.

This is why you are weighed when you go for a life insurance medical examination! The insurer knows that the risk to life increases steadily with increasing weight. Being slightly overweight is associated with a slight increase in risk, whereas being grossly overweight is associated with a serious increase in risk. Thus, the single most compelling reason for losing excess fat and achieving an acceptable body weight is to extend life.

THE IDEAL BODY WEIGHT

Fortunately, as far as health is concerned, the concept of an ideal body weight is a fluid one and should really be thought of as an acceptable body weight *range*. We can put a more precise figure on this range by using the concept of the body mass index (BMI). The BMI is a simple measurement which takes account of your age, bone structure, body shape, muscle mass, gender, etc. Using a calculator you can calculate your BMI quite simply:

- Weigh yourself in kilograms
- Measure your height in metres
- Multiple your height by itself (height squared)
- Divide your weight by your height squared
- The result is your BMI.

The formula looks like this:

$$\frac{\text{Weight (in kilograms)}}{\text{Height}^2 \text{ (in metres)}} = \text{BMI}$$

Let's take an example. Say your height is 1.74 metres, and your weight 90 kg. Multiply your height by itself: $1.74 \times 1.74 = 3.0276$. Now divide your weight (90) by your height squared (3.0276) to get your BMI, in this case 29.7.

The ideal BMI, as far as health is concerned, is anything between 20 and 25 – a reassuringly broad band. Hence, we do not need to be worried about a little excess flab here and there! A BMI between 25 and 30 is the current definition of 'overweight', and a BMI greater than 30 is defined as 'obesity'. Morbid obesity refers to a BMI of 40 or more. Now we can quantify the risk of overweight and obesity a little more accurately: a BMI of 34 is associated with a 1.5 increased mortality risk, and a BMI of 36 with a two-fold increased risk, etc. In other words, you are twice as likely to die prematurely if you have a BMI of 36! The higher the BMI, the higher the risk.

Similarly, a BMI that is too low is also associated with ill-health and a risk to life. On a global scale this is most frequently and obviously seen during times of famine. In affluent societies, an unacceptably low BMI may arise during the course of physical and/or mental illness. Perhaps one of the saddest and most frustrating examples of this is anorexia nervosa, which is defined by a refusal to maintain even the absolute minimum acceptable body weight – a BMI of 17.5. Conversely, the ideal body weight (BMI 20–25) is associated with no increased risk to health or life.

APPLES AND PEARS

People carry their excess weight in different ways. Some appear to wrap it all around their waist; others put it on their bottoms and thighs. These distributions of body fat give rise to distinct appearances. The former are affectionately referred to as 'apples', the latter as 'pears'. It would be more accurate to refer to these as android and gynoid distributions, for they are largely due to gender and hormonal

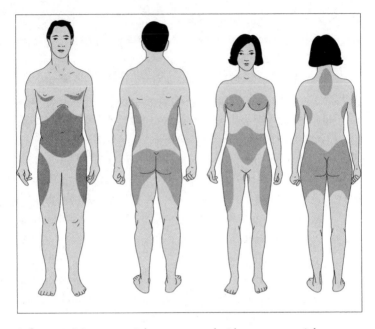

influences. Most overweight men are android; most overweight women are gynoid (see above). The differences between these two distributions of body fat are very important. The reason for this is that fat in the central (android) distribution is more metabolically active than fat in the gynoid distribution. It undergoes a more rapid turnover. The net effect of this will be seen in chapter 7. Meanwhile, we now have two more instruments with which to predict health risk, namely the waist circumference, and the waist to hip ratio.

The waist circumference is the easiest screening tool we have to identify the very high-risk patient. A waist circumference of greater than 100 cm in men and 88 cm in women is highly predictive of present or future susceptibility to chronic metabolic disease (see chapter 6). The waist/hip ratio is also a fairly good predictor of future health: a waist/hip ratio greater than 1.0 in men, and 0.90 in women, is associated with increased risk to life (mortality) and health (morbidity). Men, if your waist circumference is equal to, or greater than your hip circumference you are at particular risk. Ladies, if your waist circumference is almost equal to, equal to, or greater than your hip circumference you too are at risk.

Our life expectancy depends, at least in part, on our body weight, and on the distribution of that weight. In later chapters we will qualify this statement, we will examine how we gained weight in the first place, and we will consider the effect that overweight and obesity have on our general health and well-being.

Body weight baseline measurements

1. Measure your body mass index (BMI).* For accuracy, weigh yourself first thing in the morning, without your clothes, and after going to the toilet.

    (a) Height in metres = _____ m

    (b) Height multiplied by itself = _____

    (c) Weight in kilograms = _____ kg

    (d) My BMI is (c) divided by (b) = _____

You can also calculate what your ideal body weight range would be. This is based solely on height.

(e) For me, a BMI of 20 would be (b) × 20 = _____ kg

(f) For me, a BMI of 25 would be (b) × 25 = _____ kg

Circle your current BMI:

<23	23	24	25	26	27	28	29	30	31
32	33	34	35	36	37	38	39	40	>40

2. Measure your waist circumference. Using a flexible measuring tape, measure the waist circumference by wrapping the tape around your waist half way between the lowest rib and the wing of the pelvic bone (see diagram, page 14). If in doubt, measure the waist at its most prominent point, usually at or just above the level of the umbilicus (do not 'suck in' your stomach!). Record the measurement in centimetres.

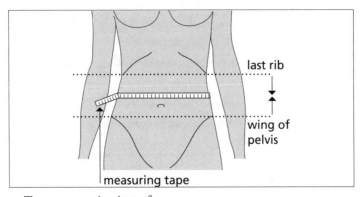

To measure waist circumference

3. Measure your waist/hip ratio. To measure your hip circumference, wrap the tape around your hips at the level of the hip bone. This is approximately where your trousers pockets would be. Record the measurement in centimetres. Now you can work out the ratio.

My waist/hip ratio

(a) waist circumference in cm = _____
(b) hip circumference in cm = _____
(c) divide (a) by (b) = _____

4. You can also assess your body weight by more conventional means. Simply find the spot on the graph opposite where your height and weight intersect.

* There is a BMI calculator at www.joefitzgibbon.ie

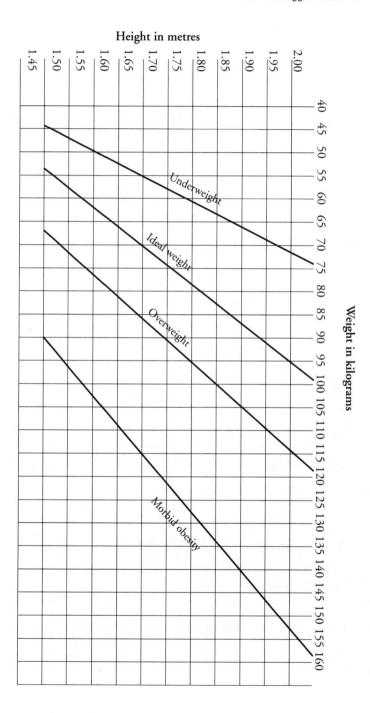

2

Understanding Metabolism

n understanding of the process of weight gain will assist us in several ways. Most importantly, it will help us to separate the simple truth about fat from the many conflicting 'theories' that have led to widespread misinformation and confusion. You will soon discover that there is no great mystery to fat, just a simple (and wonderful) physiological process. You will also find that knowledge of the mechanisms of weight gain will greatly help when it comes to the process of weight loss.

METABOLISM

We eat to sustain life. Food provides us with the basic raw materials for growth, metabolism and repair. And we need a lot of it: the average adult consumes at least one ton of food per annum! A healthy diet must provide sufficient quantities of protein, carbohydrate and fat; as well as a diverse range of vitamins and minerals. The former are referred to as macronutrients, the latter as micronutrients. As far as body weight is concerned, we are particularly interested in the macronutrients; and we will refer to micronutrients only in relation to general health. One of the principal values of macronutrients is that they provide us with energy. Food is fuel.

Our bodies are kept at a constant temperature of 37°C. To maintain that temperature requires fuel, in much the same way that heating our houses requires fuel. Our hearts beat 72 times per minute, our chests expand 22 times per minute, our intestines constantly digest food, our nerve cells communicate, our immune cells watch, our kidneys filter, and so on. Indeed, every single cell in our body is busily working away at the molecular level. All of these involuntary (not-consciously-controlled) activities are essential to life, and we refer to them, therefore, as 'basic metabolic activities'. Together they have a considerable metabolic requirement for fuel – a constant need for energy. We call this the resting, or *basal metabolic rate* (BMR). And that's *before* we start to walk around, climb the stairs, run, cycle, lift weights, wash the dishes, iron the shirts, or even sit down for a cup of tea! All of these physical activities require fuel over and above the BMR. More on this later.

Meanwhile, how can we measure your BMR? Well, to do this accurately we would have to admit you to a highly specialised metabolic unit, and that's not likely to happen. But we can learn a lot from the research that has been done in this area. As far back as the late eighteenth century, it was discovered that the life-sustaining process of metabolism, as alluded to above, could be boiled down to a fairly straightforward reaction of chemical combustion, in which oxygen is consumed and carbon dioxide is produced. Rates of oxygen consumption and carbon dioxide production may then be measured to determine the extent of chemical combustion at rest, i.e. the BMR.

In these experiments, the subject is confined to a specially designed chamber, and invited to rest by lying down on a bed. The temperature in the room is closely controlled, and the air is sampled over several hours. By this means, we can determine how much energy was used up in simply staying alive. It transpires that an average 40-year-old man uses slightly more than 1 calorie per minute at rest when awake, and slightly less (although sometimes more) than that when asleep (the concept of calories is fully explained on pages 23–4). Over the course of a day the total BMR of our subject would be approximately 1,750 calories. There is variation between individuals, however. Some people have a metabolism that is 10 per cent more efficient than the norm, and others are 10 per cent less efficient – in much the same way that some engines are more efficient than others. It is therefore more accurate to assert that our subject has a BMR of 1,750, *plus or minus* 10 per cent. It follows from this that the metabolic requirement of someone with a very efficient (energy-sparing) metabolism could be 20 per cent less compared to someone with a less efficient (energy-wasting) metabolism. This explains, at least in part, why some people are more prone to weight gain than others.

Another interesting finding from these studies is that larger people have greater energy requirements than smaller people. 'That's obvious!' you may say. 'We would expect a grown man to need more energy (food) than an infant.' And that is true: a one-year-old infant would need less than a third of the calories of an adult man. However, take two 40-year-old men and put them side by side. Notice that one of them is obese, and the other is thin. Which one do you think would have the higher BMR? Some might be inclined to indicate the thin man as having the higher metabolism in the belief that this is what keeps him thin. But the fact of the matter is that the obese man has the higher BMR! Why? Because there is more of him! The fat he carries around is not just sitting there doing nothing: it has a metabolic requirement! Energy is required to maintain it.

So, whilst we fully accept a variation in the efficiency of metabolism between one person and the next, we cannot use this as an excuse. We have to abandon the notion that 'I'm overweight because I have a slow metabolism!' The truth is that the heavier we are (or become), the higher our metabolism will rise. Indeed, we can go even further than that and assert that the BMR is *always* dependent on weight.

Research has provided us with mathematical equations from which we can estimate our BMRs. Note the crucial role of body weight in these equations. Remember, too, the variation of plus or minus 10 per cent. Why don't you calculate your BMR and enter it in the space provided . . .

How to calculate basal metabolic requirement (measure body weight in kg)

BMR (kcal/day)

Males	10–17 years old	$17.7 \times$ body weight $+ 657$
	18–29 years old	$15.1 \times$ body weight $+ 692$
	30–59 years old	$11.5 \times$ body weight $+ 873$
Females	10–17 years old	$13.4 \times$ body weight $+ 692$
	18–29 years old	$14.8 \times$ body weight $+ 487$
	30–59 years old	$8.3 \times$ body weight $+ 846$

My basal metabolic requirement is approximately:

_____ ($\pm$ 10%) calories.

It should be pointed out that our basal metabolism fluctuates somewhat during the course of everyday life, and may be influenced by our nutritional status, our thyroid function, and the activity of our nervous system. The menstrual cycle, in women, may also exert an influence; as will the states of pregnancy and lactation. Needless to say, during times of illness our metabolism can increase quite dramatically. 'Burning up with fever' is an accurate expression in more ways than one: we do burn more energy when we fight infection. However, for all practical purposes, the BMR estimated from the equation above is fairly accurate.

The BMR accounts for some 60–75 per cent of our total daily energy requirement. In other words, the biggest portion of the energy content of our food is used to simply keep us alive. The physical activities of daily life, in a moderately active person, account for between 15 and 30 per cent of our total energy requirement, and the digestion of food accounts for up to 10 per cent. That last point provides an interesting aside. The processes of eating, digesting, transporting, metabolising and storing food requires up to 10 per cent of the energy contained in that meal. This implies that the next time you eat a chocolate bar you can console yourself with the knowledge that 10 per cent of the calories contained therein are burnt off as you eat it! Sadly, the other 90 per cent could be stored as fat!

PHYSICAL ACTIVITY

We are all familiar with the concept of burning fat during exercise, but we should remember that all physical activity requires energy over and above the BMR. Obviously, sedentary lifestyles are less energy-demanding than more active ones, but even sedentary activities have an energy requirement. For example, sitting at an office desk requires some 1.5 calories per minute, and walking slowly requires something like 2.5 calories per minute. In contrast, physically demanding activities, such as nursing, farming and building, require twice or three times this amount of energy.

This introduces the concept of a *physical activity ratio*, or PAR. The PAR is a mathematical calculation of the increase in energy requirement over and above the BMR, and is expressed as a multiple of the BMR. For example, intensive athletic training may increase the energy requirement of the athlete by anything between 10 to 15 times the BMR. Thus, the PAR of intensive training is anything up to 15, depending on the work performed. This is, of course, an extreme example. Nevertheless, we must realise that all physical activity increases our energy requirement, albeit by varying amounts. Once again we can make use of research to give us some idea of the energy requirements of our more mundane activities. For instance, watching television or eating a meal increases our energy requirement by 1.1 to 1.4 times the BMR (not a lot), making beds increases it by 2.5, gardening by 3.5, etc. Clearly, the more physically demanding the work, the greater will be the PAR. Another obvious point to make is that the longer the activity continues, the greater will be the overall energy requirement to sustain it.

During the course of a typical day we undertake a variety of activities, and each one of these will have its own energy requirement. The sum total of all our activities is formally referred to as the *physical activity level*, or PAL. Health promotion experts advise us to achieve an average PAL of 1.7. From the figures given above it may seem that this should be easy to achieve. But the sad truth is that less than a quarter of all men and less than an eighth of all women (in affluent societies) are this active! Most people have a PAL in the region of 1.4.

The reason, of course, is that our lifestyles have changed dramatically in recent years. As a society, we have sedentary jobs where we used to be manual workers, we drive when we used to walk, use escalators and lifts instead of stairs, and watch television rather than take fresh air. The result of all this luxury is that we have deprived ourselves of a very natural way of burning off excess fat. This inactivity is one of the principal causes of overweight and obesity in affluent societies.

As mentioned earlier, one of the principal values of macronutrients is their energy content. The ideal diet is one which provides us with exactly the right amount of energy to meet the needs of our BMR and physical activities combined, no more and no less. We refer to this as our total energy expenditure. You can estimate your own total energy requirement by multiplying your BMR by your PAL. For example, a typical adult male, aged forty years and weighing 75 kg, with a PAL of 1.7 would have a total energy requirement of:

$(11.5 \times 75 + 873) \times 1.7 = 2,950.35$ calories per day.

If he led a sedentary lifestyle his energy requirement would be considerably less:

$(11.5 \times 75 + 873) \times 1.4 = 2,429.7$ calories per day.

During the course of everyday life we are adept at matching our energy needs with our food intake, but even small errors accumulate over time. This subject is dealt with in chapter 3, but at this stage we can make the following observations:

(i)   If we eat less than we need we start to fade away.

(ii) If we eat more than we need the excess is converted and stored as fat.

Think of it like this: fat is fuel, stored. In very simple terms, then, we become overweight because we ingest more energy than we burn.

3

The Energy Content of Foods

Food contains energy. To illustrate this fact, let us consider an example far removed from body weight. At a certain point in time the UK experienced an excess production of wheat. Rather than let it go to waste, it was suggested that the glut be used as fuel, and it was. Steam engines were stoked with wheat instead of coal, and the trains ran quite smoothly on wheat until the glut was exhausted and the system reverted to coal. It has been shown that human beings can extract almost as much energy from wheat as the steam engine could. The greater efficiency of the steam engine is due to the fact that it can burn the entire wheat package, whereas we only 'burn' the digestible parts and excrete the non-digestible remainder in faeces.

In purely scientific terms, energy is defined as the ability to perform work, and the 'unit of energy' is called a joule, after the man who first described it. In nutrition we also refer to joules (and megajoules) in terms of both our energy requirement, and the energy content of foods;

but most people are not aware of this, and would be more familiar with another unit of work, the kilocalorie. A kilocalorie is the amount of (heat) energy required to raise the temperature of 1 kg (1 litre) of water by 1°C; and a calorie is the amount required to heat 1 gram (1 millilitre) of water by the same amount. In practice most people would think in terms of calories, and so will we.

Reverting to the wheat-driven locomotive for a moment, it is clear that the calorie content of wheat could be released (by burning) to supply power to the engine. Coal, along with all other petrochemicals, also contains energy which can be released in the same way. As human beings our bodies are unable to extract the energy locked up in petrochemicals. Not only are they indigestible to us, but they are toxic to boot. The reason for even thinking along these lines is to bring home the fact that food is largely a form of energy that we can use. Food is fuel. And any fuel that is not used up, not 'burned off' if you will, must be stored somewhere. We store it as fat. It is worth repeating: fat is fuel, stored.

Not all foods have the same energy content. Some have more than others. If we were to break a meal into its component macronutrient parts we would end up with carbohydrates, proteins and fats; and each of these has its own energy content. In approximate terms:

Carbohydrates contain . . .	4 calories per gram
Proteins contain . . .	4 calories per gram
Fats contain . . .	9 calories per gram
(Alcohol contains . . .	7 calories per gram)

With the exception of alcohol, it is virtually impossible to eat a meal without all of these being present, to some extent at least. In fact, we could go even further than that and assert that it would be impossible to eat pure protein, or pure carbohydrate, or pure fat, other than under artificially engineered circumstances. It is therefore somewhat artificial to consider them separately, but it is useful nonetheless. By knowing the relative amounts of each macronutrient in a given meal (or food), and knowing the energy value of each of these, we can estimate with some accuracy the total energy content of the meal.

The important concept to grasp at this point is that all foods have energy. It does not matter to our metabolism where we get our energy from, just so long as we get it. Our bodies are able to extract energy from all of the macronutrients: be they protein, carbohydrate or fat. By way of illustration, imagine for a moment that you were shipwrecked and marooned on a desert island. The only thing you could salvage from the sinking ship was a large case of pure protein powder (which was destined for use in a science laboratory somewhere). You could survive quite happily on this food for some time! It would taste awful, and it would be nowhere near nutritionally complete, but as far as energy is concerned it would be perfectly adequate. Each gram would yield 4 calories of energy. So, if you were an average 40-year-old male, with an average BMR of 1,750 ($\pm$ 10%), and an (inadequate) average PAL of 1.4, you would have a total energy requirement of 2,450 calories per day, and this would be met by eating 612.5 (2,450 divided by 4) grams of the protein powder each day. So, what would happen if you ate more than that? You would put on weight! How? By the conversion of excess protein (energy) to fat (energy stored)!

Now imagine that you were stranded on the island, not with pure protein, but with pure carbohydrate. The very same principle would apply, namely, that pure carbohydrate would be a perfectly adequate source of energy to meet your daily needs. And because protein and carbohydrate contain virtually the same energy, we can confidently state that 612.5 g of pure carbohydrate would meet your daily requirement. So, what would happen if you ate more than that? You would put on weight and get fat, of course! How? By the conversion of excess carbohydrate (energy) to fat (energy stored).

Now imagine that you were stranded with a case of pure fat. Once again, it would meet all of your energy needs quite easily. In fact, you would need a lot less of it because fat contains 9 calories per gram: 272.2 g per day would be sufficient. What would happen if you ate more than that? The excess fat would be stored as fat.

Finally, imagine being stranded with an endless supply of alcohol! There is something of an exception here, because the amounts of pure alcohol needed to supply total energy requirements would be, *de facto*, intoxicating, with serious disruptions to metabolism in general. In everyday life, alcoholic beverages supply up to 6 per cent of the daily energy requirements of moderate drinkers in affluent societies. If that 6 per cent were in excess of the daily requirement, it would give rise in due course to the infamous 'beer belly'.

These desert island scenarios are quite daft. Perhaps it would be more realistic to think of being stranded with no food whatsoever! What would happen then? The body would burn up its own resources of energy. It would start by using the stored carbohydrate, then it would draw on fat, and finally even the protein would be used.

Carbohydrate stores would be exhausted very quickly, usually within one day. Fat stores, on the other hand, could keep you going for much longer; and if our stranded subject happened to be obese they could even last months (theoretically, at least)! Finally, as fat stores become depleted, the body would have no choice but to turn its attention to protein. The muscles and internal organs must yield their protein content to the energy demands of essential-to-life metabolic processes.

This would be analogous to burning the floorboards after the oil, coal, and gas have all been used up, and even the furniture has been sacrificed – there is just no other way to keep your house warm in the depths of winter. Such extreme nutritional poverty leads to emaciation, the classical state of malnutrition. As the energy resources are further depleted there is simply not enough energy to maintain vital metabolic functions. Immunity fails and infections take advantage; other organs and systems also fail, giving rise to much illness and ultimately death, unless the energy (and micronutrient) deficit can be corrected.

In this book we are dealing with the antithesis of emaciation, namely fatness. As you can see, we grow fat because we eat more food (energy) than we burn off, whatever the food source of that energy. This chapter attempts to impart some understanding of the fact that all macronutrients supply energy and can therefore contribute to overweight and obesity. Bear in mind, however, that fats are more energy-dense, and hence more fattening, than either proteins or carbohydrates. In fact, they are almost twice as fattening! Thus, a diet that contains large percentages of fat relative to protein and carbohydrate will be more fattening than any other possible dietary combination of macronutrients. This is the truth behind the saying that 'fats make you fat'.

It may surprise you, but overweight and obesity are correctly thought of as states of malnutrition, and as you will soon discover, they too can lead to much illness and premature death. We will deal with these in later chapters, but we should first consider the great usefulness of fat, both in our diet and in our bodies.

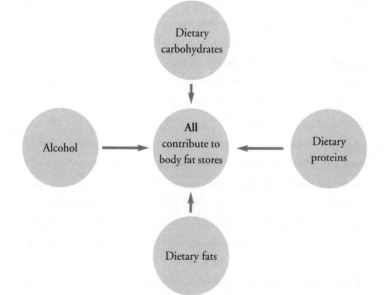

4

The Great
Usefulness of Fat

The average adult male body should contain 15 per cent fat (by weight). This truth immediately alerts us to the fact that fat serves some useful function. It must be emphasised that the reference above is to the ideal male body. This man would look slim, with no visible fat. He might look fairly muscular, but still he contains a healthy amount of fat distributed around his body. The adult female should contain even more, an average of 28 per cent fat. The extra fat in females is distributed mostly in the subcutaneous tissues (beneath the skin). The main purpose of the higher fat percentage in females is to facilitate childbearing and breast-feeding.

Clearly, we all have fat in our bodies. We refer to our fat cells collectively as adipose tissue. The difference between one individual and the next is not so much the number of fat cells they possess, but the amount of fat stored in each fat cell. A few of us have too little, some of us have just the right amount, and too many of us have too much! If 15 per cent of the weight of an average adult male is fat, what is the other 85 per cent? Quite simply, we refer to it as the 'fat-free', or 'lean' body mass. This is the collective weight of our bones, muscles, internal organs, etc., apart from their fat content.

In chapter 1, I promised to qualify the assertion that our life expectancy depends partly on our body weight. The first qualification is this: very muscular people may have a BMI above the acceptable range without being excessively fat, and without an increased risk to life! For this reason, an assessment of our percentage body fat would be more useful to us than either total body weight or BMI. Unfortunately, all attempts at such measurement have so far failed in terms of accuracy and/or convenience. In any case, we should not invoke the 'big muscles theory' as an excuse for being too heavy. The vast majority of us do not possess the muscle mass necessary to raise our BMI to this extent; and that is as true for the reasonably fit as for the sedentary. If you are in any doubt, you could always look in the mirror! These excesses of visible fat are evidence that your percentage body fat is indeed too high. Suppose, for example, that your ideal body weight is 80 kg. Fifteen per cent of this, or 12 kg, would be healthy fat. But if you weigh-in at 88 kg, you are 8 kg overweight. This 8 kg is virtually all fat, so now your total body fat is in the region of 20 kg (the original 12 'healthy' kg + the excessive 8 'unhealthy' kg). Your percentage body fat has now risen to 22.7 per cent (20/0.88), a considerable difference. This shows how easily a modest increase in weight can lead to a substantial increase in percentage body fat, and thence to health consequences.

Meanwhile, what is the purpose of fat in normal healthy individuals? We have established that fat is fuel stored. But we should not think of this as some abandoned depot, forgotten by the body. On the contrary, fat stores are metabolically highly active – much more like a beehive than a derelict warehouse. The activity is focused on the body's immediate requirements for energy. The principal role of adipose tissue is to release energy into the blood stream when available energy sources are low, and to receive and store energy when the blood levels of energy are surplus to immediate requirements. Thus, there is a constant stream of transactions taking place in adipose tissue – endless deposits and withdrawals of energy.

What is fat exactly? Tri-acyl-glycerol! Let's make it simple: the largest portion (over 90 per cent) of energy in our bodies is stored as fat. The largest portion of fat is triacylglycerol. Each unit of triacylglycerol consists of three fatty acid units (*tri-acyl-*) linked to a glycerol unit. Simply put, then, fat is composed of fatty acids and glycerol. We are equipped with enzyme systems that can break down triacylglycerol and release its component units as and when the need arises. The glycerol unit, in turn, is easily converted to glucose, and this can be used as a source of energy by all cells; whereas the fatty acids can only be used by some cells.

In health, and in the well-fed state, most of the cells in our bodies do not choose fat, protein or even whole carbohydrate directly for energy purposes. They choose glucose. This includes cells that are able to use fatty acids if they have to; if they could speak, they would tell us they prefer glucose. We can think of it like this: glucose is the main energy currency in our bodies, and all other currencies (all other forms of dietary energy) are first converted to glucose before they are used as energy. Brain cells, red blood cells, and cells in the retina (in the eye) all rely exclusively on glucose for energy, and are unable to use fatty acids. Other cells, such as muscle for instance, will use fatty acids quite happily; thus leaving what little glucose is available for those cells that cannot do without it. In summary, then, most of the cells in our bodies deal primarily with glucose, and it is only when glucose is low that we turn our attention to fatty acids. In other words, if glucose levels are adequate, there is no net withdrawal of energy from fat stores! Staying with the analogy of currency, our everyday cash transactions take place in glucose; our bank deposits are always made in triacylglycerol (fat); and our withdrawals are made in glucose and fatty acids. Finally, and only in emergencies, our protein can be used for energy after it has been broken down and converted to glucose.

It is quite clear from the foregoing that glucose has a central role in metabolism. We would, therefore, do well to study this role in a little more detail. Glucose is crucial not only in relation to our energy transactions and the weight changes that accompany them, but to the health consequences of overweight and obesity. As you will see in chapter 6, abnormal glucose levels play a fundamental part in the illnesses and mortality associated with being overweight or obese.

MORE ABOUT GLUCOSE

Glucose, in biochemical terms, is a 'saccharide', i.e., a sugar unit. Because it is a single unit, it is called a 'monosaccharide'. Fructose and galactose are examples of other monosaccharides. Some sugars consist of two monosaccharide units bound together, and these are known as 'disaccharides'. Lastly, there are sugars which consist of very long chains of monosaccharide units bound together, and these are known as 'polysaccharides'. Monosaccharides and disaccharides are simple sugars, whereas polysaccharides are complex. Sugars are also called carbohydrates, so there is plenty of room for confusion over the terminology! In practice, these terms are used interchangeably.

There are three major sources of glucose in the normal human diet. These are:

- sucrose, which is the disaccharide sugar we buy in bags (consisting of glucose and fructose)
- lactose, which is the disaccharide sugar found in milk (consisting of glucose and galactose)
- starch, which is the polysaccharide sugar (consisting predominantly of glucose units all linked together) found in almost all foods, but especially in cereal grains.

Glucose in the fed state

When these sugars are eaten, they are digested in the gut like any other food. The polysaccharides, being complex sugar molecules, are gradually broken down to their constituent monosaccharide units. Because each monosaccharide is bound to the next one in the chain, it takes a relatively long time to digest the whole polysaccharide. This ensures a gradual absorption of sugar into the blood. The disaccharides, on the other hand, need very little digesting because they only have one bond to be broken before releasing their two monosaccharide units. Finally, when sugar is ingested in the monosaccharide form, it needs no digestion at all! Ingestion of monosaccharide or disaccharide sugars will cause a rapid increase in blood glucose. This is where the concept of the glycaemic index comes from. Foods which give a rapid rise in glucose are said to have a high glycaemic index.

Glucose is by far the most important monosaccharide, so we can forget about the others, and concentrate on it alone (besides, the other monosaccharides must first be converted to glucose before they can be of any use). Glucose is more or less immediately absorbed into the blood, and taken to the liver for processing. The liver has a large storage capacity, and will hold on to about two-thirds of all the glucose ingested. In doing so, it prevents the unacceptable rise in blood glucose levels which would otherwise occur after meals. The remaining one third passes directly into the blood, and stimulates the pancreas to release insulin. Insulin then promotes the transport of glucose into the billions of cells around the body, thus providing them with essential energy, but causing a fall in blood glucose levels in the process. The liver detects the falling level of glucose, and responds to it by releasing some of the glucose it was holding on to, thus restoring the blood level to normal.

Surplus glucose, not immediately required for energy, is polymerised (linked together) and stored as glycogen in virtually all cells. However, this capacity is quite limited. Liver and muscle cells devote 8 and 1 per cent of their respective total weights to glycogen storage. This glycogen may be quickly broken down to provide glucose if the demand should arise. But once the glycogen storage capacity is saturated, the remaining surplus glucose is converted to glycerol; glycerol is then bound to three fatty acids to form triacylglycerol; and this is stored in adipose tissue as fat. Similarly, any protein or fat in our diet which is not immediately used will also be converted to triglyceride and stored as fat.

Glucose in the fasting state

The foregoing applies mostly to the fed state, where food is plentiful and we have recently eaten. So what about the fasting state? As you might expect, glucose levels in the blood are carefully controlled between meals. After all, our cells require glucose at all times, not just immediately after food has been ingested. This is achieved by the balanced interaction of:

(a) the two pancreatic hormones, insulin and glucagon
(b) the liver
(c) the stress hormone adrenaline.

The pancreas, of course, is better known for the enzymes it secretes into the intestine for the digestion of food; but it also contains two other cell types. One of these secretes insulin, and the other secretes glucagon, directly into the blood. Together, these mechanisms ensure that (i) energy is always available to cells; and (ii) glucose levels are not allowed to rise to dangerous heights, in spite of intermittent meals.

Fasting, from a metabolic point of view, starts 4 to 5 hours after your last meal! As glucose is used up inside cells, the blood glucose levels fall, and the body calls on glycogen stores to replenish them. But all of the glucose and glycogen would be (theoretically) used up within one day! The stores would be completely empty within that time. So, when glycogen stores start to become depleted the body calls on fat stores. Fat (triacylglycerol) is broken down to fatty acids and glycerol.

In contrast to the limited energy stores in glycogen, the fat stores of an average healthy male could (theoretically) keep him supplied with energy for 70 days! And considerably longer if overweight. If the fasting continues, protein will also be broken down to provide glucose to glucose-dependent cells, as already stated.

THE GREAT USEFULNESS OF FAT

Now we can see the real usefulness of fat. It allows us to eat intermittently and get on with our lives. We do not need a constant drip feed of glucose. Fat also provides us with a store of energy to draw on in times of emergency, such as during illness, for example, or when we have to skip a meal for whatever reason.

However, we are an affluent society with an abundance of available food. We probably fail to appreciate fat as much as we ought. Consider, for a moment, an entirely different situation in which food is not so readily available. When you are hungry, or even starving, you want to be able to eat whatever food is available, whenever it becomes available. The fact that you can store what you do not immediately need is a very useful function of adipose tissue. This storage facility would also have been very useful historically, especially in times of hardship. When food was available, typically during summer time after a bountiful harvest, our forefathers could eat to their hearts' content and put on a little weight in the process. They would then have had a store of energy to keep them going during the long winter months when food was scarce. Thus they would pass through cycles of modest weight gain followed by weight loss, and they would have maintained a healthy body weight year on year. Can you see what has happened in our affluence? We gain a little weight all right, but we don't lose it again! There is simply too much food available, or at least, it is available on a constant basis. We no longer face long harsh winters, or have to stretch our rations to ensure they last till spring. Thus, the little weight we gain, we keep; and then we gain a little more, and then some more again.

Other uses of fat

I should also mention that fat is useful for other reasons. In the first place, because fats are so energy-dense, it is practically impossible to obtain sufficient energy and maintain a normal body weight without some fat being present in our diet. Furthermore, some vitamins (A, D, E and K) are fat-soluble and can only be obtained by eating fats. Finally, fats are involved in cell membrane structure and function, and provide the basic building blocks for many important chemicals and hormones.

5

How is your (Fat) Balance?

You've already been brave enough to declare your BMI, so you probably have some idea of how much weight you would like to lose. Stay with the concept of energy, rather than weight, for a little longer. Fat is energy stored. With this in mind we can change the usual question from 'how much excess weight do I carry?' to the much more interesting 'how much excess energy do I store?' We have already established that both males and females have a normal healthy fat content, and that this fat can provide energy for prolonged periods if need be. But in this chapter we are interested only in our excess energy stores. So, the discussion that follows refers to the energy we carry over and above our natural reserves.

Up till now you have patiently accepted the recurring theme that fat is energy stored. You may have found this a little vague, so let's get specific. What is the precise relationship between energy and fat? To answer this, stay with the example of our average middle-aged man, with an average BMR of 1,750 and an (inadequate) PAL of 1.4. He has a total energy requirement of 2,450 calories per day (BMR × PAL). What would happen if he were to eat, say, 10 calories per day more than this? He would put on 0.5 kg in one year! You may think that an excess of 0.5 kg is very little, hardly noticeable in fact, and certainly not overweight. But if this tiny excess is repeated year after year it will lead to a weight gain of 10 kg in 20 years. And now our hapless lad is definitely overweight! This is the basis of the middle-age spread.

You may wonder how we can be so precise, so let me remind you of what a calorie is. A calorie is the amount of energy required to heat one gram of water by 1 degree centigrade. Experiments prove that 1 kg of fat can heat approximately 7,000 g of water by 1°C! In other words, there are approximately 7,000 calories in each kilogram of fat. If you prefer imperial measurements, each pound of fat contains between 3,000 and 3,500 calories. You can use this knowledge to figure out your own energy balance. Write down the following:

My current body weight (kg) = _____

The upper limit of my ideal body weight range[1] (kg) = _____

The difference between the two (kg) = _____

Multiply the difference by 7,000 = _____ calories stored

_____

[1]Height × height × 25

The result is the number of calories stored in your excess fat – and it is a conservative estimate! Now take the example of a 45-year-old woman, who is 1.63 metres (5'4") tall, and who weighs-in at 75 kg. This would give her a BMI of 28.2, which means that she is overweight. The upper limit of her ideal body weight range (a BMI of 25) would be approximately 66.5 kg.

Her current body weight	=	75
Upper limit of ideal range	=	66.5
Difference between the two	=	8.5 (75−66.5)
Multiplied by 7,000	=	59,500 calories stored in excess fat

We can take this a step further. Her total daily energy requirement (BMR × inadequate PAL of 1.4) would work out at some 2,056 calories per day. This means that, in theory, she has enough energy stored to last her for 29 days (we arrive at this figure by dividing 59,500 by 2,056)! And that's before she delves into her natural fat reserves.

Let us now examine the margin of error involved in this amount of overweight. Our subject is 8.5 kg over her upper ideal body weight range. She probably gained this weight slowly and imperceptibly over the past 20 years or so. That's 7,300 days; and that works out (roughly) at an excess of (59,500 divided by 7,300) 8 calories per day. Her total daily energy requirement was 2,056 calories; she ate an extra 8 calories per day, which represents an error of 0.39 per cent. The same is true of our earlier example. The average middle-aged man with the daily energy requirement of 2,450 calories who ate 10 calories per day over and above his needs had an error of just 0.4 per cent. So what about you? What was your margin of error over the past 20 years? You can calculate this easily by dividing your total energy store by 7,300 days. Write it down!

My margin of error over the past 20 years (in calories):
Excess energy stores (from the calculation above) =   calories
Divided by 7,300 =   daily excess calories

You can also work out your percentage error. Simply divide the number of excess calories per day by 1 per cent of your total daily energy requirement (BMR × PAL). For example, the woman above had a total daily energy requirement of 2,056. One per cent of this is 20.56. She ate an excess of 8 calories per day, so divide 8 by 20.56.

You end up with a figure of 0.389 per cent (which I rounded off to 0.39 per cent).

My percentage error over the past 20 years:

(a) calories eaten daily in excess of requirements = _____

(b) 1 per cent of my total daily energy requirement = _____

(c) divide (a) by (b) = _____ % error

The discerning reader might object to these precise figures. 'There is no such thing as a straight line in biological systems,' you may say; and I accept that. One kilogram of fat, taken from one individual person, may contain a little more or less than 7,000 calories. And other factors would come into play during episodes of weight gain, dieting or starvation which would seriously disrupt my neat calculations. But the principles of the calorie content of fat, and of the margins of error, are absolutely correct.

Eight to ten calories per day are tiny excesses, equivalent perhaps to half a rice cake, or one spoonful of muesli. But it is an excess that accumulates relentlessly over the years. It is a subtle excess, outside the realms of conscious decision-making. For this reason it is referred to as the 'passive consumption of calories'. It explains why we suddenly come into middle age and discover that we are fat! We fend off this stark and unpleasant conclusion with all sorts of explanations, but we are only kidding ourselves. 'Oh, it's just my body shape changing with age,' we say; or 'I just need to tone up' a bit. Listen, it's FAT! It got there very *very* gradually by a process of passive consumption. The excesses were tiny, but cumulative. I trust you can see that it has nothing whatever to do with gluttony or slovenliness. It has everything to do with an affluent lifestyle, and the ravages of time.

What about the very obese? Surely they have made a substantial error? Not so. Take another example, this time a 45-year-old woman, 1.63 metres tall, who weighs 108 kg. She has a BMI greater than 40, by definition severely obese. Her ideal upper body weight limit would be 66.5 kg, so she is 41.5 kg overweight. That's equivalent to an energy store of 290,500 calories. Over 20 years she has consumed 39.5 calories per day more than she has burnt off. In other words, she has eaten just half a grapefruit per day over and above her daily requirements, and that's without sugar or honey to sweeten it! Surely this cannot, by any stretch of the imagination, be construed as gluttony. And yet our society looks down on these unfortunate people. In their defence, I would like to point out that there are just four references to gluttony in the Holy Bible. Each one of these mentions gluttony and drunkenness in the same breath. This suggests to me that gluttony properly refers to a lifestyle characterised by an insatiable appetite for food and drink – quite different from the passive consumption of calories that besets our affluent lifestyle and accounts for the vast majority of the overweight and obesity problems that we see. So why do doctors and other health professionals go on and on about the importance of body weight? Because overweight and obesity have far-reaching implications for health, that's why!

Section 2

Health Effects of Overweight and Obesity

6

Diabetes

A strange thing happens as we put on weight: we become less sensitive to the effects of insulin. We don't know exactly why this should happen, but we suspect it is because insulin receptors on the cell walls are not functioning properly. Cell receptors are like keyholes. They accept the key (and only that key) for which they are built, the key turns, the lock is opened, and something specific happens inside the cell. In the case of insulin, the insulin receptor (keyhole) will only accept an insulin molecule (key). Once inserted, the key turns, the lock opens and glucose is specifically transported into the cell. Insulin has other effects as well, as we will see in due course.

In the process of gaining weight, we are exposed to increased levels of fatty acid (fats) in our blood. It is thought that these fatty acids clog the insulin receptor mechanism in some way, leaving us insensitive to the effects of insulin. To put it another way, our cells become resistant to the effects of insulin. Insulin reaches the key hole, but it can no longer turn the lock. The consequences of this can be devastating. A loss of insulin sensitivity leads first and foremost to diabetes mellitus.

There are different types of diabetes. We are particularly interested in the type that is associated with excess body weight; it is called non-insulin dependent diabetes mellitus (NIDDM). Let me explain. As the name implies, there are two main types of diabetes mellitus. One is referred to as 'insulin-dependent' and the other as 'non-insulin dependent'. Let's look at insulin-dependent diabetes first, and that will help us to better understand the non-insulin dependent type.

In chapter 4 we described the important role which insulin plays in keeping blood glucose levels normal. Insulin works by promoting the movement of glucose out of the blood stream and in to cells all over the body. Without the insulin effect, glucose entry into cells is severely restricted. Glucose levels then build up in the blood, sometimes to very high levels. This is called hyperglycaemia.

Meanwhile, cells which are dependent on glucose for energy metabolism are deprived of energy. This really is a case of 'famine in the midst of plenty' for there is ample, even excess glucose available just outside the cell wall, though it cannot find a way to get inside the cell.

Those cells that are able to, will switch their metabolism from glucose to fatty acids. Other cells may start to break down their own protein in an attempt to convert it to glucose and overcome the dearth of glucose within the cell. This effect on protein is compounded by the fact that insulin has a second action in the body: it promotes the manufacture of new protein. Thus, protein metabolism suffers twice. Firstly, protein is broken down; secondly, protein is not replaced. Before long, the end-products of protein metabolism (ketones) start to build up in the blood and permeate the whole body; they spill over into the urine and they can even be smelt on the breath.

Meanwhile, elevated glucose levels in the blood have a strong osmotic effect and cause excessive urine production. This effect may be extreme, with vast volumes of urine being passed at frequent intervals (polyuria). This in turn leads to excessive thirst (polydipsia), and to hunger. By now, our patient is very unwell indeed. He has developed diabetes. In this case, it has reached the stage of diabetic ketoacidosis – a metabolic crisis. He needs urgent and expert medical help to restore his health. Treatment consists of insulin (by injection), fluids (by i.v. drip), and correction of the acidosis.

These severe and sudden onset diabetic emergencies are most commonly seen in younger patients, but can occur in other age groups. In these situations, the diabetes has nothing to do with weight. It has to do with a primary failure of the pancreas to produce insulin, possibly as a result of viral infection in a genetically vulnerable individual, or as a result of auto-immune destruction of insulin-producing cells. This kind of diabetes always requires immediate (and long-term) treatment by insulin injection, hence the name 'insulin-dependent diabetes'. In summary, then, insulin-dependent diabetes is caused by insulin 'deficiency' and is treated by insulin replacement.

In non-insulin dependent diabetes, there is adequate production of insulin, but the body stops reacting to it in the normal way. Our cells become resistant to the insulin that is present and no longer respond to it as they should. In fact, the insulin level actually rises in this situation in an attempt to overcome the relative insensitivity. So now we have elevated levels of both insulin and glucose in the blood. In the early stages, the glucose elevation is not very high. It may continue undetected for months, or even years. But once started, the elevated glucose level will only get worse with time, particularly if weight continues to be gained. At first, the symptoms may be minimal and hardly noticed. A little more thirst, a few more trips to the toilet, or gradually worsening fatigue; symptoms that are easily put down to the stresses and strains of life – or to the underlying weight problem!

This form of diabetes is on the increase. In the vast majority of cases it is the direct consequence of being overweight! In fact, there is a virtual 'epidemic' of NIDDM occurring under our very noses. And they say that for every case in which the diagnosis is made, there is another case missed. This is hardly surprising. The increased incidence of NIDDM simply reflects the increased incidence of overweight and obesity which causes it in the first place. The problem with undiagnosed diabetes is that damage is already taking place. Early intervention would prevent many of the complications.

We can prove the link between overweight and diabetes in two ways. Firstly, take a group of healthy men (who have no family history of diabetes) and deliberately overfeed them for a while. What happens? They lose insulin sensitivity and their blood levels of insulin rise. Next, get them to lose weight again. What happens? Their insulin sensitivity is restored. Secondly, weigh every single patient who is newly diagnosed with NIDDM. What do we find? Over 75 per cent of them have a BMI greater than 25! These two findings establish beyond doubt that excess weight gain is strongly associated with diabetes. Note, also, that we are not just talking about morbid obesity or even 'simple' obesity. We are talking of all overweight, which by definition starts at a BMI of 25. Let me drive this point home another way: if my BMI is higher than 25, I am running a real and definite risk of developing diabetes. Having an acceptable body weight does not guarantee immunity from diabetes, but it does reduce my risk significantly. Genetic predisposition renders some people more susceptible than others. Hence some overweight people will escape, and some ideal-weight people will not.

Once the diagnosis of NIDDM is made, you can imagine that there is no great point in giving insulin. We have to correct the underlying cause of the diabetes. The good news is that we can do just that. In the experiment above, our healthy volunteers were able to restore their sensitivity to insulin by losing weight. Exercise also helps in this regard and we will come back to exercise in chapter 15. In some cases it will be necessary to treat NIDDM with a combination of (i) medicines that help to reduce blood glucose levels, and (ii) a low sugar diet. These measures will be needed until such time as significant weight loss has been achieved, and insulin sensitivity restored.

Incidentally, NIDDM used to be (and is still sometimes) called by other names, such as 'maturity-onset diabetes' or 'type II diabetes'; whereas insulin-dependent diabetes was also called 'juvenile-onset diabetes' or 'type I diabetes'. Furthermore, it is possible for the non-insulin type of diabetes to worsen, and turn into an insulin-dependent type.

DIABETES, DOES IT MATTER?

There are significant long-term implications for anyone with diabetes which should cause concern. I draw your attention to these, not as a scare tactic, but by way of encouragement and in the hope of motivating you to do something positive about it! You can and must do all in your power to reduce the risks.

Diabetes is a metabolic disease. As such, it has the potential to affect virtually all systems in the body. Diabetics are at particular risk of the following:

- eye disease (retinopathy) leading to blindness
- heart disease (angina)
- heart attacks (myocardial infarction)
- nerve damage (neuropathy)
- kidney damage (nephropathy)
- stroke (cerebral infarction).

How can this be? There are two fundamental problems for diabetics. These are nerve cell damage, and small blood vessel damage. I mentioned earlier that insulin is required to facilitate transport of glucose into cells. This is particularly true of muscle cells, but there are two cell types that do not need insulin in order to get hold of glucose. These are (i) our nerve cells, and (ii) the cells lining our small blood vessels (capillaries). When you think about it, this is actually a good thing. Brain cells cannot survive on anything other than glucose. The fact that they can receive glucose without the help of insulin therefore ensures their survival even when something goes wrong with the insulin mechanism. However, the down side is that glucose, when it is present in excess, can enter nerve and capillary cells at will, without regulation, and build up to toxic levels inside the cell. Nerve cells, when they are damaged by excess glucose, give rise to symptoms of altered sensation, such as pins and needles, pain and numbness. Numb skin is easily damaged, giving rise to diabetic ulcers, particularly on the feet.

Damaged capillaries cause severe disruption to the blood supply in several areas, notably the eye, the kidney, the heart, and the circulation of the lower limbs. Indeed, diabetes is the most common cause of blindness in the Western world. It is also the most common cause of gangrene leading to amputation. The diabetic heart suffers greatly in that (i) heart attacks are five times more common in diabetics, and (ii) heart attacks account for 75 per cent of deaths in diabetics. Similarly, damaged blood vessels in the brain lead to an increased risk of stroke.

It is quite clear, then, that diabetes can be a devastating disease. You cannot do much to alter your genetic predisposition to it, but you can alter your body weight and thus greatly reduce your overall risk!

7

Heart Disease and Stroke

I t is somewhat arbitrary to divide this chapter from the last for there is much overlap between the two. We are still discussing insulin resistance and high blood insulin levels. Elevated insulin levels are strongly associated with high blood pressure (hypertension); and with high levels of circulating fats, notably cholesterol and triglycerides. In fact, it is quite common to find . . .

i) insulin resistance (and elevated glucose levels)
ii) elevated blood fats (especially triglycerides and cholesterol)
iii) hypertension, and
iv) overweight

. . . in the same individual!

Whenever we find a cluster of problems in medicine we tend to think in terms of a syndrome and we look for a common underlying cause. This syndrome has been variously called the Deadly Quartet, the

Insulin-Resistance Syndrome, and the Multiple Metabolic Syndrome. *The common underlying cause is excess body weight!*

As we have seen in the previous chapter, the diabetes of overweight gives rise to significant problems of its own. But the high blood pressure and elevated blood fats spoken of here compound these effects and further increase the risk of potentially serious problems, e.g. heart disease and stroke. These are the major causes of debilitating illness and death in those who are overweight.

To understand what happens we need to back-track a little, to the normal metabolism of glucose. I would also like to draw your attention to the destiny of dietary fats – the fat content of our meals. In health, that is, in an adult male with 15 per cent body fat or an adult female with 26 per cent body fat, dietary fats are handled as follows:

- The meal is eaten.
- Blood glucose levels go up.
- Insulin is released from the pancreas in response.
- Glucose is transported out of the blood and into cells in a regulated fashion.
- The fats in our meals are absorbed in a unique way. They are 'wrapped' in varying amounts of protein to form specialised transport compounds. This is an important step because fats are not water-soluble, and if absorbed 'neat' they would clog up the system very quickly. Wrapping them in protein allows them to be carried in the blood to their final destination.
- Within a few hours of eating a meal our blood is heavily laden with these fats. So much so, that the plasma looks cloudy to the naked eye. You could even leave the plasma to stand overnight and in the morning the cream (the fatty layer) would have risen to the top!
- In health, these fats are quickly removed from our blood stream and stored as fat. Fat is energy stored.

I previously alluded to the fact that insulin has other effects apart from glucose transport. One of these effects is to *inhibit* the breakdown of fat stores. Insulin achieves this effect by inhibiting the enzyme that breaks down fat. When glucose is readily available as a source of energy, there is no need to dig into our fat reserves. The same insulin that promotes glucose entry into cells tells the fat cells to hold on to their energy stores. There is no need for them to release glucose and fatty acids into the blood when glucose is already plentiful. Furthermore, if glucose is plentiful the chances are that fats have also been recently eaten in the same meal. But to return to fat metabolism:

- As time goes by, and a fasting state is entered, the glucose levels fall.
- Insulin levels also fall in response.
- This lifts the sanction on the enzyme that breaks down fat.
- Fat is broken down.
- Glucose and fatty acids are released into the blood stream.
- Cells are able to continue functioning on these sources of energy.

What do you think might happen in states of insulin resistance? Although there is plenty of insulin about, it is unable to inhibit the enzyme that breaks down fat. Consequently fats are broken down on a continuous basis and fat levels build up in the blood. And when a meal containing fat is eaten, the blood levels rise even higher. Now we are at risk from the detrimental effects of excess fat levels in our blood.

Central body fat is particularly important in this regard. The reason for this is two-fold. Firstly, central body fat has a high turnover rate. It has plenty of fat-breaking enzymes. Secondly, the fatty acids thus released from central body stores pass directly into the abdomen, and thence straight to the liver. Once they reach the liver these free-floating fatty acids cause an increase in the production of triglycerides. Triglycerides are now incorporated into – and dramatically change the metabolic behaviour of – cholesterol in the blood. This is when all the trouble really starts. We noted earlier the importance of waist circumference and the waist:hip ratio. The larger your waist, the more central fat you have. And here is another interesting fact: we accumulate fat *inside* our abdomens, not just on the outside where it is visible! To appreciate this fact let us look in more detail at cholesterol.

CHOLESTEROL

Cholesterol is a very important molecule. Our bodies use it to manufacture the sex and steroid hormones, for example, as well as bile salts; and our cell membranes need it in order to function properly. However, we generally have too much of it. Our blood carries cholesterol in various forms. Most commonly, it is bound to protein in various ways to form lipoproteins (*lipo-* referring to lipid, or fat). We have low-density lipoprotein and high-density lipoprotein cholesterol. These names are shortened to LDL cholesterol and HDL cholesterol respectively. The former is considered 'bad cholesterol', the latter 'good'. LDL cholesterol is bad because it accumulates in tissues and causes trouble. HDL cholesterol is good because it removes cholesterol from the blood by transporting it back to the liver, thus removing it from the circulation. HDL cholesterol is not obtained in our diet; it is manufactured in the body (mostly in liver cells). It is the only way we have to get rid of cholesterol from the system.

The excess production of triglycerides that occurs in overweight dramatically alters the metabolism of cholesterol in two ways. Firstly, they make the LDL cholesterol very small and dense, and thereby much more likely to cause disease. Secondly, they change the HDL cholesterol into a less efficient form, one that is not so good at removing cholesterol from the blood. Together these changes give rise to atherosclerosis.

ATHEROSCLEROSIS

Atherosclerosis is the disease process that gives rise to blocked arteries throughout the body. It develops in the following way. Small and dense LDL cholesterol is more difficult for the body to handle. It stays in the blood stream longer than it should, and because of its small size it finds it easier to squeeze through the blood vessel wall and lodge there. Once lodged in the vessel wall it is modified further by free radical damage. LDL cholesterol thus modified is 'mopped up' by special cells before it can do any further damage, but this ability is limited. These cells become engorged with LDL cholesterol and cannot cope with the workload. The LDL cholesterol now attracts the attention of other cells which move into the vessel wall in a valiant attempt to neutralise the danger but in so doing they open the flood gates for other inflammatory (immune) cells, and even more LDL cholesterol.

Now we have a full-blown inflammatory disease underway. The vessel wall becomes cramped in the process and bulges into the lumen of the vessel. This vessel is now stiffer and narrower than it should be. Some remodelling of the vessel takes place but this is somewhat akin to Custer's last stand. The atherosclerotic plaque thus formed undergoes further degradation and attracts the attention of platelets. These stick to the plaque and further restrict the lumen of the vessel. Sometimes a clump of platelets will suddenly dislodge from the plaque and travel in the blood stream as an embolus. The embolus will travel through the vasculature until it reaches a point where it can no longer fit, it gets stuck, and the vessel is blocked. Every cell distal to the blockage is now cut off from its blood supply and will enter a state of dire emergency. Cells which are thus deprived of all support will quickly die. If, instead of breaking off as an embolus, the platelets continue to accumulate on the atherosclerotic lesion, they can eventually completely obstruct the lumen. This is called thrombosis.

Emboli and thrombi in the coronary vasculature will cause cardiac emergencies, such as angina and heart attack. Similar events in the cerebral circulation will cause stroke (other sites throughout the body may also be affected). The bigger the embolus or thrombus, the more extensive will be the damage. Unless circulation can be quickly restored to the deprived cells permanent damage will ensue.

LDL CHOLESTEROL AND HEART DISEASE

There is absolutely no doubt of a strong association between LDL cholesterol levels in the blood and the risk of heart disease. The relationship between the two is linear: for every 0.026 mmol/L increase in LDL cholesterol, there is a 1–2 per cent increased risk of heart disease. Clinical trials have established the benefit of reducing your cholesterol levels if these are too high. You may be asked to go on a specific low-cholesterol diet, but if your levels are up significantly you may need a cholesterol lowering drug. However, although the LDL cholesterol association is strong, it is not the full story. For example, why should one person with a serum LDL cholesterol level of, say, 5.2 mmol/L get a heart attack when his neighbour, who has the same level, does not? There must be other factors at play here. Genetic and environmental issues immediately come to mind as important contributors; but we may also need to pay more attention to the other fats in our blood, namely the triglycerides. Even moderately raised triglyceride levels can alter the type of LDL cholesterol, making it much more likely to inflict damage to arterial walls.

PREVENTING HEART DISEASE AND STROKE

Heart attacks and strokes are devastating illnesses, sometimes fatal as we all know. We also know that there are several risk factors apart from weight that conspire to bring an individual into these dangerous waters. Family history, for example, is important, but usually through the genetic mechanisms that affect cholesterol metabolism. This being so we can keep an eye out for cholesterol levels, and more importantly for triglyceride levels. Cigarette smoking is also an important risk factor, probably because of the free radical damage it causes to LDL cholesterol and to the blood vessel wall. Finally, high blood pressure is another factor that plays a role and that we can monitor. So what part does overweight really play? It has been estimated that overweight (a BMI greater than 25) accounts for up to 30 per cent of all fatal heart attacks! That is a very significant contribution. Once again, we cannot choose our parents, and we have to live with our genetics; but we can stop smoking and we most certainly can lose weight!

8

Other Health Problems

People who are overweight and obese have quite a burden to bear. Not only are they subject to the metabolic diseases just covered, but they are also at increased risk of many other medical problems. Some of these arise directly from the mechanical burden of carrying excess weight, and others appear to arise as a consequence of altered metabolism.

CANCER

Overweight and obese individuals are at greater risk of developing cancer at several sites. The overall increased risk is thought to be considerable. Overweight men, for example, are 1.3 times more likely to develop cancer of the prostate, and 1.5 times more likely to succumb to bowel cancer, when compared to their slim friends. Similarly, overweight women are 1.8 times more likely to get cancer of the uterus, but this figure rises to 4.5 times in the severely obese. Other cancers are also more commonly diagnosed in the overweight. These include cancers of the breast, pancreas and gall bladder. We are not sure why this should be, but the studies are consistent: excess weight puts us at risk of cancer. As always, we readily acknowledge that body weight is only part of the story, but a part of great interest to us because we can do something about it – lose weight!

ARTHRITIS

Some complications of obesity come as no great surprise. Arthritis in weight-bearing joints, for instance, is easily understood. The hips and knees were designed to bear a limited amount of weight, and being overweight puts an extra stress on the lining of these joints leading to excessive 'wear and tear'. We call this osteoarthritis. However, it is not entirely correct to say that excess weight-bearing is the cause of excessive wear. In the first place, the ankles are usually spared in osteoarthritis, and they have to carry even greater weight than the hips or knees! The hips have to carry the full weight of the torso, but the ankles have to carry the torso and the full weight of the lower limbs – so why are they not affected if it is simply a question of excess weight-bearing? Furthermore, osteoarthritis can affect non-weight-bearing joints such as the finger joints. But whatever the true cause, there is an association between being overweight and developing arthritis. Obese individuals who lose weight report a reduction in knee pain (and finger pain) early on in the course of their weight loss. In other words, pain reduction is one of the first benefits of losing weight.

Obese people are also at greater risk of contracting gout, a painful and acute inflammation of joints which affects men over the age of 40 years, and post-menopausal women. The condition is more common in affluent societies, and especially amongst those who (a) were born with a genetic predisposition to it, and (b) over-indulge in food.

VARICOSE VEINS, VARICOSE ECZEMA, DEEP VEIN THROMBOSIS

The overweight are thought to be more prone to varicose veins and deep vein thrombosis (DVT). There are other possible contributing factors, of course, including prolonged standing, dehydration, prolonged inactivity, straining at stool (constipation), etc., but we are principally concerned here with body weight.

Varicose veins are dilated, elongated and tortuous veins most commonly seen in the legs (haemorrhoids are varicose veins in the rectum). In and of themselves, varicose veins cause little trouble, but they are associated with poor circulation. This deprives the skin of its proper nutritional support leading to a loss of skin integrity. In time, the skin becomes more and more inflamed. This is a form of dermatitis variously called 'stasis' or 'varicose' eczema. The skin assumes a waxy sheen and a tanned appearance. It may also be intensely itchy. This chronic venous insufficiency, as it is called, can also lead to a complete breakdown of skin integrity, developing further into a leg (venous) ulcer. Sometimes the skin of the entire body becomes severely inflamed. In these cases the patient may be very ill and require admission to hospital.

DVT is a condition in which the blood clots in the veins, most commonly in the lower limb or pelvis. Classically, this causes a painful swelling of the calf but the real trouble starts when the clot breaks off and starts to travel. A free-travelling clot is called an embolus. The embolus travels the length of the vein until it reaches the heart. From there it is pumped into the lungs where it causes a major obstruction. This is called a pulmonary embolus. It happens to one in every thousand people, so it is quite a problem; and 30 per cent of those affected die suddenly or within 30 days of the event! Obesity is cited as one of the independent risk factors for haemorrhoids, varicose veins, and DVT: obese men are 1.2 times more likely to suffer in this regard; and obese women are 1.5 times more likely.

SLEEP APNOEA

It has been mentioned in chapter 7 that fat tends to accumulate inside the body, and not just in the visible places we are familiar with. Overweight and obese individuals accumulate fat in the upper airways, specifically in the neck. This may in turn lead to snoring, and repeated snoring may cause further changes to the structural integrity of the upper airways. The soft palate, for example, may become elongated and swollen by repeated snoring. In short, the airways become too 'floppy'. Furthermore, in some individuals the tonsils may be too large, or the lower jaw and tongue may be set too far back. The net result is that breathing becomes difficult during sleep.

'Sleep apnoea' literally means 'not breathing during sleep'. Obviously, this refers to repeated brief episodes of not breathing during sleep, rather than a total and prolonged cessation of breathing – which would result in death! There are two main reasons for a failure to breathe properly; one is mechanical and the other is neurological. In the context of overweight and obesity we are only concerned with the mechanical type of apnoea. This also happens to be the most common form. It results from obstruction in the upper airways, by the tissues that surround the upper airways.

As air is sucked in with each breath the soft tissues vibrate off each other, a sound we recognise as a snore. As the muscles relax during sleep the soft tissues collapse completely and cut off the airway. Carbon dioxide levels then build up, and oxygen levels fall. These are potentially serious biochemical events, and they trigger an alarm in the brain. The brain responds by waking up, for a split second (a microarousal), to take what we might call a 'conscious breath'. There may be hundreds of these brief interruptions throughout the night, and they disrupt the sleep pattern profoundly.

However, these microarousals are too brief to be remembered in the morning. Thus, the patients themselves are usually unaware of the problem. What they are conscious of is a vague sense of poor quality sleep, and excessive daytime sleepiness. They are prone to microsleeps throughout the day, i.e. they fall asleep on their feet, for a split second at a time, many times a day. They also complain of poor concentration, irritability, poor memory and low mood. They may experience dull morning headaches and impotence. In severe cases, the heart comes under increasing pressure and heart disease, high blood pressure and stroke may eventually ensue. Sleep apnoea affects 2–4 per cent (conservative figures) of middle-aged adults, most commonly overweight men.

Classically, it is the spouse who brings attention to the possibility of sleep apnoea. Spouses tell us that the patient snores heavily, and they describe a rather typical sequence of events.

- They hear the usual thunderous snoring (the floppy airways vibrating together).
- This suddenly stops (the airways become completely obstructed).
- Then there is what seems like an age of silence, usually about 10 seconds (the apnoea).
- This is followed by a violent gasp for air (the brain waking up for a conscious breath).
- The cycle is repeated throughout the night (severely disrupting the sleep pattern).

Patients with sleep apnoea will usually complain of excessive daytime sleepiness.

Take a minute to fill out the Excessive Daytime Sleepiness Questionnaire below. This simple instrument has been shown by clinical trial to accurately identify those who have a sleep disorder. You simply rate your likelihood of falling asleep in various situations. The ratings are on a four-point scale, with 0 representing a 'no chance' and 3 representing a 'high chance' of falling asleep. When you answer the questions, bear in mind that we are referring to your usual routine of recent weeks and months. Some of the situations may not apply directly to you. In these cases give your 'best guess' answer. Add up your score, and compare it with the graph on page 62.

We can learn several things from this graph. In the first place, scores above 9–10 are always abnormal. They are an indication of significant

QUESTIONNAIRE	**Excessive Daytime Sleepiness Questionnaire**	**Scoring Scale:**
		would *never* dose = 0
		slight chance of dozing = 1
		moderate chance of dozing = 2
		high chance of dozing = 3
	Situations	**chance of dozing**
	Sitting and reading	
	Watching TV	
	Sitting inactive in a public place (e.g. a theatre or a meeting)	
	Sitting as a passenger in a car for an hour without a break	
	Lying down to rest in the afternoon when circumstances permit	
	Sitting and talking to someone	
	Sitting quietly after a lunch without alcohol	
	Sitting in a car, while stopped for a few minutes in traffic	
	Total	**/24**

Excessive daytime sleepiness scores and associated sleep disorders

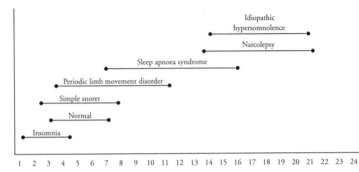

daytime sleepiness. Excessive daytime sleepiness is almost always caused by insufficient or disordered sleep. The common disorders include:

- Chronic sleep deprivation (not included in the graph)
- Restless legs and periodic limb movement disorder (PLMD)
- Sleep apnoea syndrome
- Narcolepsy (excessive daytime sleepiness with cataplexy and hypnagogic hallucinations)
- Idiopathic hypersomnolence (excessive sleep; cause unknown).

It should also be said that obese individuals may experience excessive daytime sleepiness even if they do not have sleep apnoea.

We are concerned here with sleep apnoea. All patients with sleep apnoea are encouraged to avoid alcohol and other sedatives and to avoid deliberate sleep deprivation, as these will aggravate the condition. Treatment possibilities include the well-known anecdote of changing the sleeping position from flat on the back to lying on one side, but this will only help some patients. Weight loss for the overweight and obese is encouraged, but at least 20 kg need to be shed before the sleep quality will improve. If these measures fail, then significant improvements can be secured with artificially assisted respiration. This involves wearing an oxygen mask or nasal prongs during sleep, and a machine delivers air under constant pressure throughout the night. This keeps the airway open and prevents the floppy tissues from collapsing. Special oral appliances may also be tried in an effort to achieve the same goal. The last resort is to submit to surgery of the upper airways. There are several options to consider. The removal of very large tonsils and adenoids may help some, whereas operations to reduce the size of the soft palate may help others. Finally, the more drastic step of creating a hole in the windpipe to by-pass the obstruction (a tracheostomy) is reserved for patients with very severe disease who fail to respond to other measures.

FERTILITY

There is an association between obesity and infertility, although not a straightforward one. Some studies have suggested that overweight women have trouble conceiving, but others have failed to show this. What is consistently found is that obese women who also smoke are much less likely to conceive than non-smokers; so fertility depends on a number of factors, not just weight. Obesity is also an independent risk factor for early pregnancy loss. Polycystic ovary syndrome is as much a cause of obesity as a result of it and is dealt with in chapter 9.

To increase your chances of having a successful pregnancy:

■ Achieve and maintain an acceptable BMI.
■ Reduce your intake of tobacco, alcohol and caffeine.
■ Ensure optimal nutrition.

GALL STONES, GALL BLADDER DISEASE, KIDNEY STONES

Obese men and women are at increased risk of developing gall stones. These are often silent but if they obstruct the gall bladder they can cause acute abdominal pain requiring emergency admission to hospital. They can also cause chronic inflammation of the gall bladder requiring surgery. Research suggests that being overweight also predisposes to kidney stone formation, which may be extremely painful.

ACCIDENT PRONENESS

Being overweight or obese is also a risk factor for accident proneness, and particularly for broken bones. This reflects the fact that the obese are usually (but by no means always) unfit. They don't partake in sporting activity, and consequently they are less 'light on their feet'. If they stumble they are more likely to fall. They haven't got the reflexes to save themselves. Another contributing factor in relation to accidents is the change that occurs in the centre of gravity. In obese individuals the centre of gravity is abnormally forward, especially if they have a big tummy. This is a relatively unstable position and more likely to result in a fall. The fact that the obese are also susceptible to daytime sleepiness increases their proneness to accidents.

LUNG FUNCTION AND RESPIRATORY DISEASE

The lung function of obese people is impaired. We have already seen this in relation to sleep apnoea, but this is true of all overweight individuals, not just those who have the full-blown sleep disorder. The weight of their fat is constantly bearing down on their chest wall. The effort required to expand the chest is great and the work the respiratory muscles have to perform is doubled. Some estimates have put the reduction in lung capacity to 60 per cent of normal – a highly significant impairment. The most obvious manifestation of reduced lung capacity is shortness of breath, and surveys reveal that shortness of breath is a significant problem for many, especially the elderly. Think about it. Every little task requires a conscious effort to breathe. The debility that ensues is associated with poor functional ability (needing help with the activities of daily life), a restricted lifestyle, depression and anxiety. Furthermore, reduced lung capacity sets you up for recurrent chest infections. You can avoid all of this by achieving and maintaining an acceptable BMI. Another early benefit of weight loss is a feeling of increased lung capacity, more breathing power!

SKIN

The overweight are prone to intertrigo: a red itchy rash caused by fungal infection. These infections most commonly occur in warm and sweaty skin folds, such as under the arms and breasts, and in the groin. The reason for this is that the offending fungus thrives in such conditions.

Stretch marks are broad pink bands of scar-like skin that rather suddenly appear on the thighs, buttocks, abdomen, breasts and back. Females are more commonly affected. Stretch marks are associated with teenage years, but also with rapid weight gain, obesity or rapid weight loss(!). They are also well known to occur during pregnancy. No treatment is necessary and they tend to become less noticeable with time.

Benign warts (papillomas), and hyperpigmentation of the skin (acanthosis nigrans), especially in the skin folds of the neck, axillae and groin are also more common in the obese.

FATIGUE

The foregoing amounts to quite a burden for the overweight. It is even more of a problem for the very obese because all these conditions tend to be worse with increasing weight. The simple activities of daily life require a greater effort from the overweight. After all, they have a greater body mass and reduced reserve. The overweight frequently complain of feeling tired all the time, and those who successfully lose weight enjoy an early return of energy. In fact, the fatigue of severe obesity can be very profound and may even mimic the fatigue of chronic fatigue syndrome.

SURGERY

The overweight and obese have more difficulty during and after surgical procedures.

- It can be difficult to find a vein to take blood and administer an anaesthetic.
- The anaesthetic is diluted throughout a greater body mass and the dosage is more difficult to control.
- Respiratory function is further decreased.
- There is greater pressure on nerves during the operation.
- The surgeon has greater difficulty working through fat.
- There is greater difficulty mobilising post-op.
- There is an increased risk of DVT and pulmonary embolism.

Summary of health problems associated with overweight

It may be helpful at this juncture to take stock of your own health, and specifically of your own weight-related health issues. How many of the following weight-related conditions do you have/have you had?

- Diabetes mellitus (non-insulin dependent), and its complications: ❏
  - Eye disease ❏

- ● Heart disease ❑
- ● Nerve damage ❑
- ● Kidney damage ❑
- ● Stroke ❑
- ■ High blood pressure (further increases the risk of heart disease and stroke) ❑
- ■ High blood cholesterol or triglyceride levels ❑
- ■ Ischaemic heart disease (from atherosclerosis in coronary arteries) ❑
- ■ Stroke (from atherosclerosis in cerebral arteries) ❑
- ■ Cancer (especially of the breast, uterus, prostate and colon) ❑
- ■ Arthritis (especially hips and knees) ❑
- ■ Varicose veins ❑
  - ● Leg ulcers ❑
  - ● Varicose eczema ❑
  - ● Haemorrhoids ❑
- ■ Deep vein thrombosis ❑
  - ● Pulmonary embolus ❑
- ■ Sleep apnoea syndrome ❑
  - ● Excessive daytime sleepiness ❑
  - ● Headache ❑
  - ● Impotence ❑
- ■ Infertility ❑
  - ● Poor outcome pregnancy ❑
- ■ Gall stones ❑
  - ● Gall bladder disease ❑
- ■ Kidney stones ❑
- ■ Accident proneness ❑
  - ● Broken bones ❑
- ■ Poor lung function ❑
  - ● Shortness of breath ❑
  - ● Infections ❑

- Stretch marks (from obesity, or from rapid weight gain *or loss*) ❑
- Fatigue ❑
- Social marginalisation and discrimination ❑
- Poor self-image and esteem ❑
- Depression ❑

Remember, you can reduce your risk of all of these by losing even a little excess weight!

Section 3

Causes of Weight Gain

9

Medical Causes of Weight Gain

Much is said about the medical causes of overweight and obesity. We say things like 'It must be my hormones', or 'It's in my genes!' But if we were honest with ourselves, we would acknowledge that what we are really looking for is the ultimate excuse: 'There is a reason for my being fat and it has nothing whatever to do with what I eat!' We want the world to know that it is not our fault, and perhaps we want to shirk a little of the responsibility. The truth is that less than 4 per cent of all cases of overweight and obesity are due to such medical causes, and the rest of us are fat because we eat too much! However, I trust that you have left the guilt behind in chapter 5: the vast majority of us have become fat because of the passive consumption of calories over time – nothing to do with gluttony or slovenliness.

Of course, you may strongly suspect that there are other factors at play in your particular case, such as your constitution or genetic make-up. You may also suspect that you have a food allergy or some such condition which has caused your excess weight. We will examine each of these in due course. Meanwhile, and for the sake of the few who do have a medical cause for their weight gain, let us briefly look at the most common causes.

THE THYROID

The most common medical cause for weight gain is an underactive thyroid gland. The thyroid is located in front of the voice box (larynx) in the neck. It produces thyroid hormones. We do not know exactly how these exert their influence but we do know that they speed up the metabolism throughout the body. They are particularly important in childhood for normal growth, mental development, and a successful passage through puberty. In adult life they are essential for regulating metabolism, including the metabolism of the brain, heart, intestinal tract, etc.

The main thyroid hormones are thyroxine (which we abbreviate to T4), and tri-iodothyronine (which we abbreviate to T3). The T4 is converted to T3 outside of the thyroid gland by a series of enzymes. This is an important step because T3 is far more active than T4. As you can tell by the name (iodo-), iodine is an important constituent of the thyroid hormones. Inadequate supplies of iodine in the diet will lead to a functional thyroid deficiency, and iodine replacement restores full thyroid function. The thyroid gland actively takes up iodine from the bloodstream, and responds to low iodine levels by increasing its size, giving the classical goitre – a thyroid swelling in the neck. Iodine deficiency is rare nowadays, except in areas where the soil content of iodine is depleted. The addition of iodine to table salt in many countries has gone a long way to eradicating this problem.

In health, the thyroid gland is regulated by the brain, and this is how it 'knows' how much hormone to produce. Specifically, the pituitary gland secretes a hormone called thyroid stimulating hormone (which we abbreviate to TSH). TSH travels in the blood to the thyroid gland and provides the correct amount of 'stimulation', and hence the correct amount of T4 and T3 are produced. To complicate matters further, the pituitary is also regulated! It will release TSH only in as much as it is 'told' to do so by another hormone (TSH-releasing hormone) which is produced in the hypothalamus (see diagram below). Finally, there is a feedback loop from the body to the brain which lets the brain 'know' whether there is enough thyroid hormone around or not. If there is sufficient, the level of TSH drops back a bit; if there is a lack the TSH level moves up a notch. This is all very technical information but the main point is simple: the thyroid gland is regulated by a very sophisticated system in the brain.

Meanwhile, let us come back to our principal concern, namely the relationship between thyroid disorders and weight. The thyroid may become underactive (hypothyroid) or overactive (hyperthyroid), and both conditions may affect weight! We would expect anything that lowers our metabolism to result in weight gain, and anything that speeds it up to cause weight loss.

Hypothyroidism

The symptom complex of hypothyroidism leads to a gradual slowing of general metabolism, which in turn leads to the following:

- mental sluggishness
- depression
- fatigue
- weight gain
- intolerance of cold
- sluggish bowel function (constipation)

- sluggish heart rate (slower heart rate)
- sluggish reflexes
- dry skin
- menstrual irregularities
- hair loss
- hoarse voice, and other alterations in voice (particularly noticed by singers who can no longer reach the higher notes)
- puffiness of the face and legs (myxoedema)
- hypothermia (falling body temperature) and coma, in extreme cases
- also in extreme cases, a rare form of mental illness associated with severe hypothyroidism called 'myxoedema madness'.

Causes of hypothyroidism

Hypothyroidism may result from disruption to any part of the pathway from the hypothalamus to the thyroid gland itself. Most cases are idiopathic (we-don't-know-the-cause) failures of the thyroid gland itself, others are caused by autoimmune destruction of thyroid cells (in which the immune system 'attacks' the thyroid gland in the mistaken belief that it is 'foreign' rather than 'self'). In rare cases the problem has to do with failure of the stimulating system to work effectively.

Hyperthyroidism

As you would expect, the symptoms of hyperthyroidism are almost the opposite of the symptoms of hypothyroidism. There is a general increase in metabolism leading to . . .

- mental 'overactivity', restlessness, or anxiety and other emotional symptoms
- tremor (the shakes), especially in the hands
- fatigue (paradoxically)
- weight loss
- intolerance of heat

- overactive bowel function (diarrhoea)
- overactive heart rate (faster heart rate, and sometimes palpitations)
- very brisk reflexes
- excessive sweating
- in some cases, protruding eyes, giving a staring appearance (exophthalmos).

The control of thyroid function

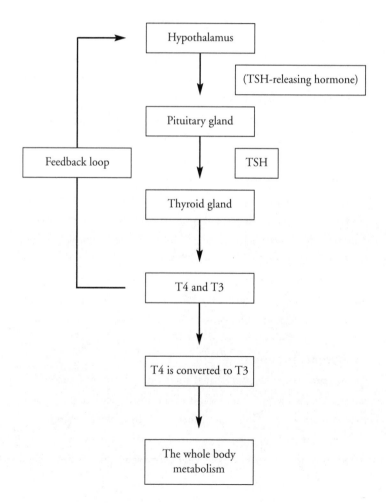

The diagnosis of thyroid disease

There are several laboratory tests which assess thyroid function. For example, we could measure T4, and we could reasonably assume that T4 levels will be lower than normal in hypothyroidism and higher than normal in hyperthyroidism. This is generally true in clinical practice. However, as in all biological systems, there is a range of normal levels. Thus a level of 60 nmol per litre of blood would be normal for some people, but others would need 160 nmol. That's quite a range. So if we measured *your* T4, and found that it was 80 nmol/l, how would we know that this was a normal level *for you*? We wouldn't! To get around this problem, we can ask your brain what it thinks! And specifically, we can ask your pituitary gland. If your TSH level is normal, then we could assume that 80 nmol/l was sufficient *for you*. If, on the other hand, your TSH level was elevated we could safely assume that 80 nmol/l was not sufficient for you. Your brain is sending out more TSH in an attempt to get the thyroid to produce more T4.

The thyroid tests may be affected by medicines, pregnancy, other illnesses, surgery and/or nutritional disturbances. But apart from these isolated cases they are reliable. In fact, the TSH level is thought to be so reliable that many laboratories use it alone to screen for thyroid function. A normal TSH is said to 'invariably mean normal thyroid function'. In hypothyroidism the TSH level can reach for the sky; in hyperthyroidism it may be undetectable. The treatment of thyroid disorders is said to be successful when the TSH and T4 levels come back within the normal range.

A thyroid argument

Some patients are convinced that their thyroid gland is underactive even when the thyroid blood test is normal. It is theoretically possible that they are correct, but only if they have *many* of the symptoms of hypothyroidism, and not just by virtue of the fact that they have one possible symptom – excess fat! Being overweight, then, is not a good enough reason to take thyroid hormone. In fact, there are potentially serious health risks associated with taking excess thyroid hormone, so be guided by your doctor in this regard.

POLYCYSTIC OVARY SYNDROME (PCOS)

PCOS is a relatively common, although poorly understood disorder affecting up to 7 per cent of women of childbearing age. It is characterised by hormonal imbalance: testosterone is produced to excess, oestrogen production is erratic, and there is resistance to insulin. As you can imagine, excess testosterone and unpredictable oestrogen levels are not desirable in a woman: they lead to 'masculinisation'. The symptoms include:

- menstrual irregularities
- acne
- unwanted hair growth (hirsuitism)
- failure to ovulate and conceive
- prominent weight gain (in 50 per cent of cases).

As mentioned above, PCOS is associated with insulin resistance. This is true even in lean women. In other words, the hormonal disturbances occur *before* the weight is gained, and that is why PCOS is classified as a cause (rather than a result) of weight gain. However, overweight and obesity have a synergistic effect in PCOS – they make matters worse.

The insulin resistance of PCOS increases the risk of metabolic disease such as diabetes, high blood pressure, high cholesterol level, elevated triglycerides and heart disease. The insulin resistance of overweight and obesity also increases the same risks, a double whammy effect. There is evidence for the benefit of weight loss in PCOS. We could go even further and assert that weight loss is part of the successful treatment of PCOS: it may improve hair growth, skin quality, menstrual pattern and fertility; it would also help to prevent the later complications of diabetes and heart disease.

The diagnosis of PCOS is made on the basis of the symptoms present, together with an ultrasound scan of the ovaries (showing a cystic appearance) and a few blood tests. The cystic appearance of the ovaries reflects the numerous follicular cysts which are being continuously stimulated but which never mature to release an ovum.

CUSHING'S SYNDROME

Cushing's Syndrome is caused by excess cortisol (steroid) production in the adrenal glands (just above the kidney on each side). It may also be caused by taking steroids, such as may be necessary (and life-saving) in the treatment of some diseases. In health, cortisol helps the body to respond to stress. It does so by a variety of mechanisms including a powerful effect of the metabolism of glucose.

The production of cortisol, like the production of thyroid hormone, is controlled by the pituitary gland. The pituitary releases a hormone (abbreviated to ACTH) that stimulates the adrenal to secrete cortisol, and cortisol exerts a negative feedback on the pituitary to reduce the secretion of ACTH. Thus balance is maintained in the system. Too much cortisol production leads to changes in all of the tissues and organs of the body, resulting in Cushing's Syndrome (after the doctor who first described it in 1912).

Sometimes a pituitary tumour secretes vast quantities of ACTH – which drives the production of cortisol to very high levels. At other times ACTH is produced by other tumours in the body, with the same effects. Occasionally, a few cortisol-producing cells in the adrenal gland throw off their submission to ACTH and spew out excessive amounts of cortisol in an unregulated fashion. But whatever the underlying cause, excess cortisol will lead to the following symptoms:

■ Weight gain, especially on the abdomen, face, neck and upper back. This distribution of weight is very much along the lines of central obesity. Weight gain on the face and upper back give rise to classical appearances of 'moon face' and 'buffalo hump'

■ Weakness and wasting of the muscles in the arms and legs, especially in the proximal part of the limb (shoulders and thighs). This may be noticed by the patient who could have difficulty using these muscle groups, such as when climbing stairs for example

■ Thinning of the skin, easy bruising and stretch marks

■ Acne and hirsuitism

■ Male pattern baldness (more of a problem when it occurs in women)

■ High blood pressure

■ Fatigue, depression and other mood changes

■ Diabetes: with excessive thirst and frequent urination

■ Menstrual abnormalities

■ Osteoporosis, especially if untreated.

Not everyone who shows these symptoms is suffering from Cushing's Syndrome. However, it is important to diagnose Cushing's Syndrome because it needs to be treated, or more correctly, the underlying cause needs to be treated. The initial diagnosis is made by a relatively simple blood test. Unexplained elevations in cortisol should be further investigated by a specialist.

HYPOTHALAMIC OBESITY

I include hypothalamic injury because of its general interest value. We have seen (above) that the hypothalamus communicates with the pituitary, and the pituitary communicates with other glands, e.g. the thyroid and the adrenal amongst others. We have also seen that glands such as the thyroid and adrenal provide feedback information to the hypothalamus and pituitary. A fascinating thing happens when the hypothalamus is damaged by injury or disease: there is a *dramatic* increase in appetite.

Most commonly, the affected patient will display intense food-seeking behaviour and will be unable to stop eating until substantial weight is gained. After the initial weight gain, the appetite 'normalises' again and the patient maintains the new (heavier) body weight. Sometimes the food-seeking behaviour (craving) is very specific for certain foods, leading to food fads (somewhat like the strange cravings reported by some expectant mothers). All of this suggests that the hypothalamus has a preset gauge for appetite and body weight, both of which can be disrupted by disease. The issue of appetite is addressed in chapter 12.

DEPRESSION

Depressive illness is a common disorder. It is characterised, in its simplest form, by pervasive feelings of low mood. Our susceptibility to depressive illness is determined by several factors, including our genetic make-up (family background), environmental stresses, and the biochemical well-being of our brain cells. Sadly, depression is still a taboo subject in our society and we are often reluctant to face up to it in ourselves. This is particularly true of men. Consequently, we resist any attempt which the doctor makes to diagnose depression. This is a pity because in so doing we deprive ourselves of effective treatment. Weight gain can be part and parcel of a depressive illness.

The following table contains a list of the principal symptoms of what doctors call 'major depression'. Ask yourself, over the last two weeks (or longer), have you experienced the following:

How do I know if I am depressed?	**Scoring Scale:** Yes = 1 No = 0
1 Pervasive feelings of low mood	
2 Loss of interest and/or pleasure in most activities	
3 Loss of appetite (and weight), or overeating (and weight gain)	
4 Insomnia or excessive sleeping	
5 Psychomotor retardation: movement and speech are very slow. Or psychomotor agitation: constantly restless and agitated, pacing, unable to sit	
6 Fatigue: this may be profound and debilitating. Simple activities may be very difficult to perform	
7 Feelings of worthlessness and guilt	
8 Difficulty concentrating and making decisions	
9 Recurrent thoughts of death, with or without a plan for suicide	
Score	**/9**

If you have ticked either 1 or 2 (or both), and have a total score of five (or more), you are suffering from major depression. Clearly, if you are feeling depressed but haven't scored five points you would still be well advised to consult your doctor for a chat. You may well have a less severe form of depressive illness.

There are other mood disorders, of course, and these may present differently. Of particular interest to us in relation to body weight is a depressive illness called 'atypical depression'. Atypical refers in this case to an unusual form of depression, in which patients complain of depressed mood together with increased appetite and sometimes marked weight gain. They are also excessively sleepy, they have feelings of leaden paralysis, and they tell us that they have become very sensitive to rejection by others. Effective treatment restores mood, sleep pattern, energy levels, and normalises the appetite. Anti-depressants may cause a modest initial weight gain in some individuals, but this is a small price to pay for a cure and can be addressed when recovery has been secured. Bear in mind also that anti-depressants have been used successfully in the treatment of weight loss!

A WORD ABOUT MEDICINES

Patients frequently ask their doctor whether a prescribed drug will cause them to gain weight. The truthful answer is that some of them do, but usually to a limited extent only. The most obvious weight-gaining drugs are the steroids, as mentioned above, especially if required in high doses and for prolonged periods of time. Antipsychotic medicines are also well known to cause weight gain. But other drugs, particularly those that work on brain cells or hormonal systems, can potentially alter appetite and/or metabolism sufficiently to cause a noticeable weight gain.

Examples of medicines that may cause weight gain

Medicine	Used in the treatment of . . .
Steroids	Inflammatory conditions
Contraceptive steroids	Family planning
Beta-blockers	High blood pressure
Insulin	Insulin-dependent diabetes mellitus
Sulphonylureas	Non-insulin dependent diabetes mellitus
Tricyclics	Depression
Sodium valproate	Epilepsy

Remember that . . .

■ The benefits of treatment would always outweigh the disadvantage of the weight gain.

■ Alternative drugs may be used in certain cases.

■ The principles of weight gain, maintenance and loss, as described in this book, hold true for any weight gain that occurs in conjunction with medicines.

■ Fat is still energy stored, and it can be burned off!

Other Causes of
Weight Gain

The medical causes of weight gain addressed in chapter 9 account for a tiny proportion of all cases of overweight and obesity. Only 4 per cent of overweight individuals will fall into this category. The rest of us will have to look elsewhere for an explanation of our weight gain. We have already established that the cause of weight gain and obesity in the vast majority of cases is a combination of two factors, namely excess calorie intake and inadequate calorie expenditure. This is an absolute biological truth, but it is also a little simplistic and therefore a little unfair. We need to ask, 'Why do *I* end up with a positive energy balance, when others around me do not?' As it happens, there are several powerful factors that conspire to make us gain weight. These include our psychosocial environment, genetic make-up, lifestyle, sleep patterns and dietary habits.

ENVIRONMENT

We have previously seen how individuals vary in terms of their energy efficiency. Some are more efficient than others when it comes to energy metabolism and are thereby at greater risk of putting on weight and getting fat; whereas the less efficient appear to 'waste' some of their energy and remain thin. The difference between any two people in this regard could be as high as 20 per cent. What accounts for the variation? Clearly there must be a constitutional element at play. Research has provided some clues but we are still a long way from having all the answers.

One consistent finding is that individuals who were of low birth weight are more likely to be overweight as adults. The apparent paradox disappears when we consider the reason for low birth weight: inadequate foetal nutrition. The growing foetus was exposed to a relatively harsh environment in the womb and nutrition was not as good as it could have been. The theory is that the developing baby responds to this challenge by adopting fundamental metabolic changes. This in turn leads to changes in how the baby handles food. These food/energy-handling changes are so deeply embedded that they remain with the person for ever, making him or her susceptible to weight gain in later years when food becomes more plentiful. In simple terms we could think of this as a 'learned' increase in energy efficiency. The infant was not genetically programmed to react in this way, but is certainly programmed to do so now.

Another observation of interest is that being thin as a child is no protection from becoming overweight or obese in adult life. In fact, some studies suggest that thinner children (not just low birth weight babies) become fatter adults! However, overweight children also have a tendency to remain overweight into adult life.

Other environmental factors known to predispose to weight gain include lower socio-economic status, and the size of one's parents.

Relative poverty in a wealthy society contributes to overweight through its effects on food choice. Some foods may be cheaper and may satisfy the family's hunger, but they are not necessarily healthier. Poor families can afford less dietary variety; and have a lower consumption of wholegrain foods, fruit and vegetables. They also have a greater prevalence of physical inactivity. Members of low-income families are at greater risk of heart disease, high blood pressure, cancers, respiratory and digestive disorders, as well as obesity.

The size of one's parents is a more difficult issue to clarify. In the first place we can say with absolute certainty that fat does run in families. But we cannot say why. Is it because children inherit the same genes as their parents and the genes make them fat? Or is it that children learn (bad) dietary and exercise habits from their parents? The answer is probably a little of both.

GENES

Twin studies show that overweight and obesity in adult life are directly influenced by genetic make-up. This can be shown by comparing the body weight of identical and non-identical twin pairs when these have been brought up together or separately (this sort of comparison helps us to distinguish genetic from environmental factors). Similarly, studies of adopted children suggest that they are much more likely to become obese if their biological parents were obese, even if their adoptive parents are lean. Once again, this suggests a genetic influence on body weight.

The risk of 'passing on' our weight problem to our children has been calculated. It is the same risk we inherited from our parents and it takes both genetics and environment into account. The bottom line is this: daughters whose mothers are obese are eight times more likely to become obese themselves (compared to their friends who happen to have thin mothers); sons and daughters are four times more likely to become obese if their father is obese. These are highly significant increases in risk. It would be of great interest if we could find a purely genetic basis to this heritage, but we cannot. Some excitement is expressed from time to time when a gene linked to obesity is discovered but the probability is that purely genetic (single gene) factors account for very few cases of obesity. The vast majority are due to a combination of genetic and environmental factors. That said, many experts in the field of obesity research believe that genetic factors are by far the more important. Some studies suggest that *the genetic contribution to obesity may be as high as 70 per cent.*

Please note this, however. If you come from an overweight family you are not thereby doomed to fatness, but you will have to work harder to avoid weight gain. Even if you are genetically programmed to put on weight easily, you will not put it on if you do not eat more than you burn off.

LIFESTYLE

Another assertion we can make with absolute certainty is that lifestyle also directly affects body weight. Lifestyle, in this context, refers to work- and leisure-related activities. Studies have shown that occupations involving light levels of physical activity, such as sitting at a desk, are strongly associated with weight gain over time. The amount of overtime we accept is also relevant because it increases the amount of time we spend at our desks, and keeps us away from other physical activities. Even jobs which were traditionally more physically demanding have been taken over by labour-saving devices. Research suggests that those who are engaged in physically demanding jobs are twice as likely to remain slim. Put another way, if you are in a sedentary job you are twice as likely to get fat! This is true whether your job is stressful or boring. You may consider your job to be the most stressful on earth, and it may well be, but that doesn't change the fact that it is sedentary! Energy burned at work has nothing to do with mental exertion; it has everything to do with physical activity – or the lack thereof. Mental activity may be tiring, but it is not energy-demanding.

The same decline in exertion has crept into other areas of our lives. We have electric mixers and squeezers, and washing machines. We drive to and from our places of work. We drop the children to school and pop down to the shops – in our cars. And of course we watch television. People who watch television for four or more hours per day are 2.4 times more likely to be obese than those who watch less than 1 hour per day. You may recognise this person as the proverbial couch potato. But let me state the obvious: four hours would be from 8 pm to midnight! I'm sure many of us fall into that category. People who spend all day at a sedentary job and then collapse in front of the television for the evening are at great risk of becoming obese. There are two reasons for this: the physical inactivity of sitting, and the fattening effect of the meals and snacks we eat whilst viewing.

SLEEP PATTERN

As a society, we have reduced our sleeping time by 20 per cent in the past one hundred years. We have also increased our work- and travel-load by an average of one full month per annum. The result is that we now have an epidemic of sleep deprivation, with 65 per cent of adults admitting that they don't get enough sleep! What they may not realise is that people who fail to get their full quota of sleep are more likely to put on excess weight. *Even one hour less than basic sleep requirements per night will result in noticeable weight gain over time.*

The other symptoms of sleep deprivation are:

- fatigue
- poor concentration and memory
- poor task performance
- difficulties with complex thought
- unreliable decision-making
- excessive daytime sleepiness
- accidental sleep episodes
- irritability, anxiety, depressed mood
- stomach problems (indigestion and heartburn)
- menstrual irregularities
- high blood pressure
- weight gain
- frequent infections
- muscle pains.

DIET

Our diets have changed in several ways in recent years. We have increased our consumption of confectionary and we have come to rely more and more on convenience foods, such as prepared meals and snacks. These foods have high fat and sugar contents. Take-away meals and fast-food also tend to be high in fat. They may be quite delicious but they do little to satisfy the appetite – you could just keep eating them! Although not filling, they are fattening.

SUMMARY

So, what makes us fat? The answer is simple, if stark. Overweight is caused by an excess of calorie intake over calorie expenditure in people who . . .

- are genetically predisposed to weight gain
- were brought up in overweight families
- cannot afford to make healthy food choices
- work in physically undemanding jobs
- watch too much television
- do not get enough sleep
- do not take enough exercise.

11

Does Food Allergy make me Fat?

There has been much discussion in recent years on the role of food allergy in relation to overweight and obesity. We have been systematically swamped by a flood of disinformation centred on the erroneous claim that obesity is a disorder caused by food allergy or intolerance. We have been offered so-called blood tests which claim to diagnose our food allergies or intolerances, and we have been promised that once we stop eating the foods to which we are intolerant we will lose our excess weight. We need to spend a little time examining these claims.

Let me clearly state at the outset that overweight and obesity are not caused by food allergy or intolerance! They are the result of eating more energy than we use, and the surplus energy is stored as fat. However, there is one grain of truth in the food intolerance story that is worth noting. Patients with food intolerance may (strangely) crave the very food to which they are intolerant. As they succumb to their food craving they consume more calories than they need, and they store the excess as fat. Even so, it is still erroneous to claim that the intolerance is making them fat. It is not. Their excessive eating is. What they need to address is the craving.

FOOD CRAVING AND INTOLERANCE

Food addicts crave a particular food, and they feel unwell if they do not get a regular supply of it. They sub-consciously gravitate towards the culprit food because they somehow 'know' that it will make them feel better. If they miss a 'dose' they will experience several withdrawal symptoms: headache, muscle pain, fatigue and mood changes are common. Eating another dose will temporarily relieve their symptoms but they have to increase their consumption to keep their symptoms at bay. They are on a slippery downward slope, and their health will gradually deteriorate over time. This may be a new concept for many readers, so let me tell you about a real-life case whom we shall call David.

CASE HISTORY

David came to see me at the age of fifty-two years. He told me about his long struggle with rhinitis, fatigue, low mood and anxiety. In addition, he suffered from weekly migraine headaches. His dietary history was informative. He had already discovered that yogurt and cheese caused headache, so he avoided them. However, he still drank a lot of milk. He volunteered the fact that milk helped him to sleep – so much so that he could not sleep without it! Furthermore, if he had to go without it for any length of time he became restless, agitated and anxious. Drinking it again immediately relieved his feeling of tension. Drinking larger quantities actually depressed him, and made him feel fatigued – but he prefered to be depressed and fatigued than anxious and restless!

These were the classical features of a food intolerance/addiction cycle. David's intolerant symptoms were: fatigue, depression and migraine. His withdrawal symptoms were restlessness, agitation and anxiety. He would never enjoy good health as long as he remained in this vicious circle. On my advice, he stopped consuming milk, and he suffered the *transient* withdrawal symptoms of anxiety and restless agitation. These gave way within a week, or so, to a sense of well-being.

FOOD CRAVING AND OBESITY

The foregoing raises the inevitable question: are people who overeat doing so because of a hidden food intolerance? The answer to this is 'yes' – but only in a small minority of cases as the following example shows:

CASE HISTORY

Noreen, a forty-year-old mother of two, came to see me with a life-long history of headaches. She also complained of rhinitis, sinusitis, generalised aches and pains, ankle swelling and obesity: she was three stone overweight. After a 14-day wash-out period, during which she ate the Low Allergy Diet (see appendix 1), her symptoms were very much improved. She had no headache, her nose was dry, her ankles slim, and she had lost a half stone in weight (mostly fluid loss). She continued to lose weight throughout the re-introduction phase. Not only did she identify the foods responsible for her headaches, but she also identified which foods gave her cravings for more food ('the crazy hungries', as she called them). In her case, these were: wheat, sugar and soy. As long as she avoided these she was able to lose weight 'effortlessly' – and without craving. If she did eat them, on the other hand, she found herself on an uncontrollable binge. She lost three stone in as many months, and she is virtually headache free.

If you are craving a particular food, avoid it completely for seven to thirty days. In so doing, make sure that you exclude it in all of its different forms. For example, a dairy-free diet would have to exclude: milk, skimmed milk, cream, ice cream, cheese, yogurt, milk chocolate, whey, casein, caseinates, lactalbumin, lactose, and any processed food, or recipe, which contains these. You may find that this relatively simple step is sufficient to provide lasting relief from symptoms (if you have any), and from craving. Of course, if you do exclude a food from your diet, make sure you have not left yourself short of important nutrients. Get professional advice if in doubt.

Please note. Noreen was obese because, over the years, she had eaten more energy than she burned off, and the excess energy was stored as fat. She lost weight because she burned off more energy than she ate, over a relatively short period of time. Obesity is *not* an allergic disease. If food intolerance makes you crave, you are likely to eat more and *that* is what makes you put on the weight!

FOOD ALLERGY AND INTOLERANCE

Hippocrates (460–359 BC) was the first physician to describe adverse reactions to food. He said, for example, that although cheese is an excellent food for most, the smallest piece could make some people ill. He had no idea *why* cheese made some people ill, only that it *did*. His approach was, therefore, simple and pragmatic. He made his diagnosis on the grounds of clinical observation alone: if the symptoms under investigation were relieved by avoiding a certain food, and returned again whenever that food was eaten, he would have advised his patient not to eat that food again. The essence of this truth was later captured by the Roman poet Lucretius (94–55 BC) with the simple words: 'One man's meat is another man's poison.'

The term 'allergy' did not come into use until early in the twentieth century when an Austrian physician (von Pirquet) first coined the phrase to describe the serious and sometimes fatal (anaphylactic) reactions, which certain children had to vaccination injections. They had developed what he called an 'altered (*allos*) reaction (*ergo*)', or *allergy*, to the horse serum contained in the vaccines.

Immediate allergic reactions to food

The nature of these immediate reactions was not fully understood until the discovery, in the 1960s, of a specialised protein within the immune system, called immunoglobulin E (IgE). IgE was identified as being responsible for initiating the cascade of allergic events which occur in susceptible individuals once they have been exposed to their allergens (an allergen being any substance – eaten, inhaled or touched – which provokes an allergic response).

IgE-mediated events are called Type 1 allergic reactions. Well known examples include hay fever (allergy to pollen), urticaria (itchy rash), angioedema (swelling of the soft tissues), and asthma (constriction of the airways). The main feature of Type 1 allergies is that they usually produce an *immediate reaction*; so much so that patients have often made their own diagnosis before they see the doctor: 'Every time I eat eggs, I break out in a rash!'

Because of the speed of these reactions, there is seldom any dispute over the diagnosis. Furthermore, it may be confirmed objectively by both skin and blood tests. The skin test is quite simple and may be carried out, on the spot, in the consulting room. A small drop of the suspected allergen is placed on the forearm, and the underlying skin is pricked with a lancet. If a wheal (a red itchy lump) develops at the site within ten minutes or so, the patient is said to be allergic to that substance. The blood test, on the other hand, is carried out in the laboratory where a quantitative measurement of IgE is made, and where the allergens against which the IgE is directed are identified. For example, if the blood is found to contain significant amounts of IgE directed against egg, then that patient, without a shadow of doubt, is allergic to egg. Strangely, the patient may not yet have symptoms when exposed to egg, in which case the allergy is described as latent, or dormant. But the potential for an allergic reaction is very much present.

It is thought that somewhere between 1 and 2 per cent of the population suffers from Type 1 food allergy. A small number of these are exquisitely sensitive to their allergens. They can experience dramatic, frightening and sometimes life-threatening reactions (anaphylaxis) after even the slightest allergen exposure.

Delayed reactions to food

The best way to develop this concept of food intolerance is through a case history of another patient, whom we shall call Carmel. Here is her story.

CASE HISTORY

Carmel was a 48-year-old teacher who had a miserable life, dogged as it was by constant illness. The day she came to see me was a relatively good day, she explained, but she was plagued with symptoms even as she spoke. She was tired all the time, she had no energy, and she had one sore throat after another. 'I've even got one now,' she protested, in obvious discomfort. She took a moment to massage her throat, and continued with her story. 'My bowels are giving me gyp, and I have pains all over my body, and –', she hesitated, as if she had suddenly remembered something. She just sat there for a while gazing at the floor, her mouth still ajar in silent mid-sentence. Then, rather nervously, she raised an inquisitive eyebrow in my direction. No, I did not think she was mad, I reassured her; and I asked her to tell me more.

It quickly became clear that Carmel had a multitude of symptoms, apparently unrelated. She had pains in her muscles and joints; her fingers and ankles were often swollen; she had mouth ulcers, bloating of the abdomen, constipation, abdominal pain and an itchy bottom; her sleep pattern was all over the place, her concentration was poor and her libido was low. Furthermore, her skin had 'gone to pot', especially just before a period. She had other premenstrual symptoms as well: her breasts were sore and she was particularly cranky for a week or so leading up to a period. As is so often the case, Carmel's medical investigations had drawn a blank, and she had been told that she was 'just depressed'. But Carmel would have none of it. 'Look', she said, 'every time I eat wheat my throat flares up, and when I eat sugar I get depressed. What I want to know is, could it be an allergy?'

Could it be an allergy?

Now there's a question that needs to be answered, for if Carmel does have an allergy, or several allergies, she could expect to find relief from her symptoms by avoiding the thing(s) to which she is allergic. Carmel's skin and blood tests would be negative for allergy. However, it would be quite wrong to leave it there. As we've said, blood tests can only show IgE allergies; they do not reveal other kinds of allergy or intolerance. This being the case, Carmel was put on the Low Allergy Diet. She was advised to eat ten prescribed foods for a period of ten days. By the tenth day she felt better than she had done for years. All of her symptoms, without exception, had disappeared. When she expanded her diet again she reacted adversely to many of her staple foods. To cut a long story short, Carmel had multiple food intolerance.

POLYSYMPTOMATICS

Carmel is not unusual – there are many like her who suffer for years on end with puzzling and debilitating symptoms. They have been on the merry-go-round of negative investigations, they have tried various medical treatments, and ultimately, they are at risk of being dismissed. Some of them are labelled neurotic, or anxious; others are told they are depressed, and a few are said to be hypochondriacal. They can see the poorly disguised heart-sinking look on their doctor's face when they present with yet another baffling symptom, and another entry into the case notes which, at this stage, are as thick as a telephone directory. Many of them will give up going to their doctor altogether for fear they will be considered 'mad'. The true nature of their illness lies buried in a jungle of *apparently* unrelated symptoms, and it lies there, hidden for years, until someone finally decides to look for it! It must be said that some of us *are* neurotic and anxious, and many of us *do* suffer from depression and/or hypochondriasis. We must also recognise that these disturbed mental states do give rise to physical symptoms! It is important therefore to keep an open mind in all of this. But my plea is that psychiatric diagnoses should only be made in the presence of a positive history of psychiatric illness; and they should never be used to fob off symptoms that are otherwise difficult to solve. The most common mistake in medicine is to assume that an illness is psychological when it isn't! The symptoms of food intolerance are a classical example of this.

TWO SCHOOLS OF THOUGHT

As you can see, we have two conflicting schools of thought in relation to food allergy. The first relies heavily on objective tests, and maintains that 'if we cannot show the *mechanism* of an allergy (by skin-prick or blood test), then it's not an allergy'. The contrasting view is empirical, and much more comprehensive. It depends, not on theory, but on what we call clinical observation and experiment. 'If you get a symptom from an "otherwise harmless" substance, you are (to put it simply) allergic to it.' In this case, it does not matter whether we can understand the mechanism; it simply matters that we observe a symptom.

The strength of the first position is that it is built on 'hard science'. But herein also lies its weakness. As you can imagine, it is very reassuring to have a reliable test which gives objective evidence of allergy. It makes the job a lot easier! However, we cannot dismiss a suspected allergy on the basis of our present inability to 'prove it' in the laboratory. To do so would be to fall headlong into a scientific trap – a dark place where otherwise brilliant minds are restricted by the limitations of their machines. The purely scientific approach to allergy tests will lead to some patients being told that they are *not* allergic when, in fact, they *are*!

Conversely, the broader proposition is founded on the art, rather than the science of medicine. Once again, herein lie strength and weakness together. It is strong because it will consider greater possibilities; it will not dismiss what it cannot understand and, consequently, will not easily 'miss' an allergy. It is weak because it cannot always prove the truth of its own diagnosis, and because it is prone to all the variables of human nature. In particular, it is vulnerable to the placebo effect: a mysterious, beguiling and often potent human response to the power of suggestion. In this case, some patients will be told that they *are* allergic when, in fact, they are *not*!

This may sound academic, but it does explain why there is so much confusion in relation to food allergy. Personally, I have a great deal of sympathy with the first viewpoint, but I am also swayed by the everyday language of my patients. If they think they react to something, they tell me they're 'allergic to it', and they care not a whit whether I can understand it, measure it or explain it!

The fall-out

One of the dangers of strongly held opposing medical views is that we can lose sight of our patients in the process of argument. Many patients have become disillusioned with what they perceive as 'medical tunnel vision' and have turned elsewhere for help. By virtue of its neglect, the medical profession has inadvertently flung the door open to the widespread use of quackery. Unqualified (and unregulated) persons have set themselves up as 'allergists', and have driven the 'allergy bandwagon' rough-shod across every unexplained symptom, including overweight and obesity. Innocent patients are told that they are allergic to various foods on the basis of unscientific and unreliable 'tests', such as vega machines, kinesiology, radionics, etc. I know of one quack that can supposedly make a diagnosis over the phone: he asks the patient to hold a piece of hair against the telephone, and he swings his pendulum over the receiver at the other end of the line! It should come as no surprise to hear that patients are often given erroneous, and sometimes even dangerous, advice.

'But I had my allergies "tested" in such a manner,' you might protest, 'and when I stopped eating certain foods I lost a ton of weight!' Okay, so you stopped eating how many foods? You went on a diet, right? You drastically cut down on your food intake and you lost weight. Surprised? You shouldn't be. There is no mystery in it! You lost weight because, over a period of time, you consumed less energy than you burned off. In other words, you dipped into your fat stores and depleted them.

'But when I stopped eating certain foods I got better and lost symptoms, not just weight!' Fine. You stopped eating certain foods and you lost symptoms. In that case, you possibly do have food intolerance, but the *method* of diagnosis is not thereby validated. Nor is the assertion proved that your weight was caused by food intolerance! In these cases I do not dispute the possible diagnosis of food intolerance, but I do most assuredly dispute the methods used to make the diagnosis. Patients who have their allergies 'tested' in this way are usually told to avoid the following foods: wheat, dairy produce, eggs, yeast, and a few others like chocolate, coffee and citrus fruit. If those suspected of food intolerance were to avoid these foods, at least 25 per cent of them would get better. Why? Because these are the most commonly eaten foods in the European diet, and it is the most commonly eaten foods which most commonly cause allergic or intolerant symptoms! Americans, for instance, would have to add peanut and maize to this list (because these are significant in the American diet), and the Chinese, for the same reason, would need to pay more attention to rice and soy! Furthermore, if you avoid all of these foods you will automatically and drastically reduce your intake of calories. If you do not eat bread, biscuits, cakes, confectionary, ice cream, chocolate, sauces, etc., you will certainly lose weight.

To put an indefinite blanket exclusion on all these foods is usually unnecessary even in those who are food-intolerant. The chances are that only one (or perhaps two) of these foods were causing symptoms, and all the others are safe. With this in mind, patients invariably experiment to see what they can get away with, but because their food challenges are not properly conducted they fail to accurately identify their culprit foods. Apart from the social nuisance of a restricted diet, there is also the danger of nutritional deficiency, and doctors have been left (on more than one occasion) to pick up the pieces of such disasters.

Please note, I do not wish to discredit alternative medicine in all of this. Numerous patients have received lasting benefit from its practitioners, many of whom have had to make good the mistakes of clumsy orthodox doctors! My plea – and this would be shared by genuine practitioners of alternative medicine – is that it be practised by persons qualified to do so, who understand all of the issues involved in health care, and who are aware of the long-term consequences of their treatment regimes.

SYMPTOMS AND MECHANISMS OF FOOD INTOLERANCE

Let us now take a closer look at the symptoms and mechanisms of food intolerance. Symptoms that may sometimes have a food intolerance component include: fatigue, migraine and other headaches, irritable bowel syndrome (bloating of the abdomen, constipation and diarrhoea, stomach cramps), indigestion, itchy bottom, inflammatory bowel disease, asthma, sinusitis, muscle pains, arthritis, eczema, hives and swellings, mouth ulcers, fluid retention, excess weight and mood changes. We do not fully understand what happens in the body during these (delayed, non-IgE) reactions but we do have some idea of the mechanisms involved. Let us take a brief look at some of these . . .

1 Pharmacological activity of food

Some food reactions are the result of powerful natural substances present in food. These chemicals exert drug-like effects in our bodies. We refer to this phenomenon as 'false food allergy'; false, only because it looks like an allergy, and is not. Here are a few examples:

- *Caffeine, an alkaloid drug.* The most widely used foods with pharmacological activity are tea and coffee. An excessive consumption of caffeine may give rise to diverse toxic symptoms: anxiety, irritability, headaches, tremor, sweats, palpitations, insomnia, restless legs, nausea, vomiting, abdominal pains, lethargy, drowsiness, depression and rhinitis.
- *Histamine-containing foods.* High levels of histamine occur naturally in some foods. This chemical is involved in allergic reactions. Histamine-containing foods include: fermented cheeses and other foods, sausages, tinned foods (especially

tinned fish and herrings' eggs), sauerkraut and spinach. These foods, when eaten in excess and/or in combination, can cause:

- flare-up of eczema
- headache
- hot flushes
- urticaria
- angioedema
- abdominal pain
- thirst
- shock (rarely).

■ *Histamine-liberating foods.* Some foods do not contain histamine, but they release histamine from mast cells in the body. This is a direct effect that does not involve IgE. Histamine-liberating foods include egg white, fish (especially shellfish), tomato, chocolate, pork, pineapple, strawberry, papaya and alcohol. They can also cause histamine symptoms.

■ *Vasoactive amines.* Vasoactive amines are also natural components of food. They have a drug-like effect on blood vessels (vaso), making them dilate. This gives rise to blood vessel headache (migraine). His*amine* is one such amine. Others include phenylethyl*amine* from chocolate (50 g is enough to cause trouble); and tyr*amine* in cheese, yeast extract, pickled herrings, banana, broad beans, liver, sausage and alcohol.

■ *Alcohol.* Alcohol is an interesting food. Apart from its universal inebriating effect and its vasoactivity, it blocks enzyme pathways, has a diuretic effect, irritates the lining of the stomach, and contains various food derivatives (and additives) to which some people are allergic.

2 Enzyme deficiencies

Food is digested by special enzymes in the gut, and further broken down by enzymes in the blood. Enzyme deficiencies will give rise to symptoms by allowing a build-up of particular food components in the gut or in the blood. One example that we should all be familiar with is our relative intolerance to onions. We do not have the enzyme necessary to digest the sugar in this food. High levels of sugar then reach the large intestine where they are fermented by resident microbes. Onions also contain a smelly disulphide. Excessive consumption of onions will therefore lead to smelly flatulence!

Enzyme deficiencies may be more idiosyncratic, however. Lactose, for example, is the sugar found in milk. Some infants are born with a lactase deficiency, the enzyme by which we digest lactose. Lactose therefore builds up in the gut causing a watery diarrhoea, and even collapse in some infants. Adults may acquire a transient lactase deficiency, especially after a bout of gastroenteritis, after intestinal surgery, or as a complication of other bowel disease. Milk consumption in such circumstances will also cause diarrhoea and related symptoms. Many other enzyme deficiencies have been identified, some of them causing serious health effects until they are diagnosed and treated by a lifetime of dietary avoidance. PKU (phenylketonuria) is probably the best known of these: every infant is checked for this at birth with the heel prick test.

3 Hormonal activity of foods

Food intolerance may also arise from foods that contain opium-like proteins. These include wheat, dairy produce and possibly maize. This may be linked to enzyme deficiency, for the proteins should be broken down by enzyme activity in the gut, and later in the blood. Symptoms known to be associated with opium-like proteins include mood and behaviour disorders, irritable bowel syndrome and water retention.

4 Toxins in food

It is hardly necessary to mention that some foods contain toxic chemicals that must be adequately degraded during cooking if they are not to cause trouble. Kidney (and other) beans, for example, should be soaked overnight and boiled for 90 minutes to break down the toxin therein. Abdominal cramps are the penalty for failing to take this precaution.

5 Sugars in food

Toddlers' diarrhoea has been linked to the consumption of apple and other fruit juices. The mechanism here is, once again, fermentation of undigested and unabsorbed sugars in the large intestine. Other symptoms include abdominal discomfort, flatulence and borborygmi (those gurgles you hear coming from your bowels). Sugar malabsorption may also affect adults.

6 Other components of food

Vegetables, like fruit, contain indigestible sugars, such as raffinose, and may cause a similar fermentation reaction. They also contain other active components. Flavone compounds, for example, are known to affect intestinal motility. This leads to abdominal distension and discomfort in susceptible people. Cabbage is notorious in this regard. Another fairly common problem is fatty food intolerance. Fats are digested by bile from the gall bladder. They can cause a great deal of trouble for patients with gall bladder disease.

7 Mechanisms for weight gain?

You will notice that there has been no mention of weight gain in the above discussion on mechanisms. There is no evidence whatever that food intolerance alters fat metabolism, for example. We still store and burn our energy stores as before. The fact that we might be allergic or intolerant to a particular food does not alter the energy content of that food! An apple is still an apple, whether it gives me a migraine or not, and its 70 calories are still 70 calories. The fact that I get migraines from apples does not, in any way, alter the nutritional qualities of the apple! For instance, I do not get any more or less than its 70 calories. Nor are these calories handled any differently by my body: they go through the very same metabolic pathways as all my other dietary calories. So how can food allergy or intolerance make you fat? They can't! But food intolerance can make you crave; and craving makes you binge and bingeing makes you fat.

'But we all crave foods!' you may say. Not true. Only some of us do. And those of us who do accept it as part of our normal appetite and eating pattern. That is why we expect everyone else to experience the same desires. If you are one who craves foods, you will want to know if your craving is related in some way to food intolerance. The clue is that food-intolerant craving is associated with other symptoms of food intolerance. If craving and its consequences (overweight) are your only complaint then forget about the intolerance story. If on the other hand, you suffer from irritable bowel syndrome or migraine, etc., then you may well have food intolerance; and that increases the chances of your craving being related to intolerance.

How do I find out if I have food intolerance?

The most reliable method for diagnosing food intolerance is the Low Allergy Diet. This involves a 'wash-out' phase, followed by the sequential re-introduction of foods. Ideally, this should only be done under the supervision of a medical doctor with a special interest in food allergy and intolerance, but many people are able to conduct their own investigation. The principle of the Low Allergy Diet is that all symptoms caused by food will cease when you stop eating the offending food. At the outset we do not know which food or foods are responsible for symptoms (if any), so we exclude everything you regularly eat. This is the so-called 'wash-out' or 'detox' phase. Foods are then reintroduced one by one to find out which ones were causing all the trouble. The dietary investigation will take approximately six weeks to complete. It is fully described in appendix 1.

12

Hunger and Appetite

Hunger is a need for food. We feel it as a physical discomfort that comes on after a period of fasting. The sensation starts off as one of mild distress, but it may become stronger and quite unpleasant if allowed to continue. Hunger will cause you to seek food – any food; and the discomfort will be relieved by eating. Appetite on the other hand is more of a desire than an absolute need for food. It may be increased by hunger, but it may not be as easily satisfied by eating. Appetite is what influences our food choice. It may determine our preference for sweet over savoury, for example. At its worst, appetite can cause you to crave food, even when you are not hungry. Appetite is what helps us to enjoy our food.

Eating is always a pleasant experience. Our brains respond to the thought, sight, smell and taste of food, whether actual or anticipated. And we will keep eating as long as the pleasure persists. The pleasure wanes somewhat as we approach the point of 'fullness'. This process is called satiation. It is associated with an increasing desire to stop eating, or rather an inability to continue eating. Once satiation is complete we enter a state of satiety. This is a complete inhibition on further eating and it signals a period of fasting – however short or long. This hunger/eating/satiation/satiety/fasting cycle is the main physiological regulator of food intake. However, it is an extremely complex process and subject to numerous influences, including the physiological, psychological and sociocultural.

If we had an 'ideal' hunger/satiety regulating system in place we would all subconsciously eat the right amount of food to supply our energy needs, no more and no less; and we would all have an ideal body weight. The problem is that satiety is often elusive. Some unfortunate people never feel full, and many more have to enhance their satiation by consciously telling themselves to 'stop eating or you'll get fat'. A few lucky individuals habitually reach satiety when they have ingested the appropriate amount of food and they stop eating without a conscious thought. So then, what are the factors that influence satiation and satiety? Let us take a more detailed look at the process of eating and subsequent feelings of fullness.

Firstly, the brain sends a message from the hunger centre and food-seeking behaviour is initiated. The mouth starts to water (salivate) in anticipation. Then . . .

The mouth:	Takes food into the body, chews it, mixes it with saliva, and initiates the swallow reflex. The act of chewing and tasting is pleasurable, and the pleasure centre in the brain is stimulated in the process.
Saliva:	Lubricates food, and contains digestive enzymes which start to work on the starch component of food straight away. We produce in excess of 1 litre of saliva every day.
The gullet (oesophagus):	Accepts the swallow reflex and carries food down to the stomach.

The stomach:	Hunger contractions cease with the arrival of food, and distension begins. The stomach stores and churns food with its own juices to form what is called chyme. Chyme is then released, bit by bit, into the small intestine. As the stomach distends further it gives rise to unpleasant sensations of fullness and hormones are sent to the brain through the blood stream to tell the satiation centre that enough food has been ingested.
The small intestine:	Receives food from the stomach, bile from the liver, and digestive enzymes from the pancreas. This mixture then travels at a rate of 1 cm per minute, thus facilitating the absorption of water and nutrients along the entire and considerable length of the small intestine. The arrival of chyme in the small intestine stimulates the release of hormones which also exert an effect on the satiation centre.
The large intestine (colon):	Accepts food from the small intestine, absorbs some water and nutrients, and stores and lubricates the waste matter (faeces) until a convenient moment for disposal.
The anus:	Prevents faeces from dribbling by its muscular (sphincter) tone.
The stool:	The whole process of digestion and absorption is so efficient that less than

The stool *(cont.)*:	one fifth of all the material entering the small intestine is eventually expelled in the stool. The smell of the stool comes from the bacterial products present therein. The normal frequency of bowel movements is quite broad, ranging from three times a day to twice a week.

As you can see, food arriving in the stomach gives rise to physical, chemical and hormonal signals. We feel immediate relief from our hunger pangs, and as time goes by we begin to feel nicely distended. As the meal progresses, the gastric distension becomes an inhibitory sensation and hormones are released to tell our brain that sufficient food has been ingested – we begin to feel full. The satiety centre in our brain (which is located in the lateral hypothalamus) will now try to reduce food intake. But these satiating messages are not the only messages clamouring for attention in our brains! There are other, sometimes conflicting messages coming from our fat cells, our endocrine system and our peripheral nerves. These may drive the hunger centre (in the ventromedial hypothalamus) to make a push for further food ingestion. And that is before we even consider the psychosocial messages: the nice food, the variety of food, the good company, the wine, the party atmosphere; or, indeed, the loneliness, the depressed mood, the comfort obtained from eating, etc. These may all override the messages of satiation and allow considerable over-eating.

The composition of a meal also affects satiation. Glucose, protein and fats will all exert some influence on our feelings of hunger and fullness. For example, the brain and liver can detect when glucose levels begin to fall and they stimulate increased food intake. When glucose levels rise, as they do after a meal, they help the brain to feel full. Complex carbohydrates (with a low glycaemic index) are much better at satiation than refined simple sugars (with a high index). In addition, the insulin response to glucose exerts an independent regulating effect on the brain which makes it feel full. Proteins are the most satiating of all foods. There are several suggestions as to why this should be so. One theory is that they alter neurotransmitter levels in the brain and exert their effects in that way. Serotonin, for example, is a major brain chemical which is made from tryptophan, an amino acid found in protein. Another suggestion is that protein is filling because it is toxic. We don't want too many amino acids floating around in our blood stream at any one time. These are controversial theories but the point is clear: proteins exert an independent effect on satiation which has nothing to do with their energy content. Fats are the most energy-dense and yet they are the least satiating of the macronutrients. They also require the least metabolism: they can be stored almost as they are eaten. These properties make fats very fattening. The most filling foods, then, are those that have a relatively high protein and carbohydrate content.

The main reason for eating is to ensure adequate energy for the activities of daily biological life. The hunger/satiety cycle helps us to regulate our food/energy intake, and most of us do so quite accurately over a lifetime. However, the fact that we are built to store excess fat suggests that satiation was never meant to stop us from periodic 'over-eating'. We subconsciously err on the side of over-feeding rather than under-feeding. In times past we never knew whether or when the next meal would arrive. We have seen, in chapter 4, how useful this capacity of energy storage has proved through the ages in helping us through times of food deprivation. The problem for us today, in a society where food is abundantly available all the year round, is that we cannot rely on satiation alone to regulate food intake. As long as our affluence continues we will need to foster some degree of conscious choice in terms of *what* we eat and *how much* we eat.

Our appetite is influenced by many factors, including the following:

■ We eat more in the evenings than in the mornings.

■ We eat more at weekends.

■ We eat larger meals when in the company of partners and close friends.

■ We eat smaller meals when in the company of business contacts.

■ We eat larger meals when eating out in restaurants.

■ We eat larger meals when the food is free (someone else pays for it).

■ Women eat at least 10 per cent more when eating with a male friend.

■ Stress, boredom, anxiety and elation all increase food intake.

■ Thirst and hunger before a meal increase food intake.

13

Food Cravings

Food cravings are difficult to define. They have little to do with hunger, that is, with the absolute need for food. They are related to appetite in as much as the pleasure of eating is anticipated. But they go far beyond normal appetite into the realm of strong urges and associated distress. Researchers have used several methods to define craving. They speak of the strength of the urge, the level of difficulty in resisting eating, and the feelings of anxiety that come when you cannot lay hold of your craved food. Craving is also characterised by marked increases in the speed of eating; and by negative feelings before and after the eating episode.

In some cases the craving seems to reach addiction proportions, at least in terms of food-seeking behaviour. Take for example the following anecdote of a woman who woke in the middle of the night with a craving for chocolate. She searched the house but found none. She got dressed and drove into the village but the petrol station was closed. She drove on to the nearest town and finally found a retail outlet. She bought several bars of chocolate and wolfed the first one down whilst sitting in the car before heading home again. She ate a second bar on the way home, and a third bar when she reached home. She thought she would feel better, but she only felt bad about herself.

This may seem like a fairly severe example of food craving, but all food cravers will recognise shades of themselves in this story. Surveys suggest that a quarter of women and an eighth of men will have experienced significant craving for food, at least once a week, every week, over the past 6 months. Both groups are likely to indulge their craving, but the women are likely to do so with more negative feelings, such as guilt or shame.

The amount of food/energy ingested during a binge can be substantial. It is quite easy to eat our total daily calorie requirement in one (moderate) binge. It also transpires that cravers have a large appetite at all times, not just when they go on a binge. So it is easy to see how cravers can quickly become overweight. Craving is a complex psycho-biological phenomenon. We understand very little of it as yet. However, there are some contributors to craving that are worth pointing out.

POSSIBLE CONTRIBUTORS TO CRAVING

Smoking cessation

Stopping smoking is a terrific positive step for health gain, but it is also a well-known risk time for weight gain. If it's the chewing that helps, try (non-fattening) nicotine gum rather than food.

Food intolerance

Craving may sometimes be related to food intolerance, in which case other symptoms of food intolerance will also be present.

Sleep disorders

We have already seen the effect of chronic sleep deprivation on food intake – it increases substantially and results in notable weight gain. The sleep-deprived person will binge, consciously or subconsciously, in the futile hope of getting an energy boost, and shaking off sleepiness. Other sleep disorders can also be associated with food cravings, possibly because of disrupted hypothalamic function. In these cases other features of a sleep disorder will also be present.

Diabetes

This is associated with increased appetite and thirst, especially when undiagnosed or poorly controlled.

Pregnancy

Some women only ever experience food cravings during pregnancy.

Premenstrual syndrome

About 50 per cent of women who crave chocolate or other sweets do so just before a menstrual period. Attempts have been made to ascribe this to subconscious nutrient-seeking behaviour. Magnesium, copper and the pharmacological effects of chocolate have all been cited. The truth is that chocolate tastes nice. It seems to have the perfect blend of texture (carbohydrates and fats) and taste. As a food, it cannot be surpassed for pleasure. It therefore has an appreciable effect on our pleasure centre. The cyclical nature of premenstrual craving may result from the low serotonin activity that affects some women at this time of the month. It is associated with depression.

Hypothalamic injury

The satiation and hunger centres are located in the hypothalamus. Hypothalamic injury is fortunately rare, but may follow brain injury, stroke, or other disease. This rare disorder is included deliberately to remind us of the biological aspect of appetite and craving.

Psychological causes

Some argue that food cravings should be understood solely in terms of their psychological context in which cravers know that they should not be eating this 'naughty but nice' food. They try to stop eating it, but become all the more preoccupied with food as a result.

BINGE EATING DISORDERS

Bulimia nervosa is an eating disorder characterised by binge eating and compensatory measures to lose weight. A typical binge would last less than two hours. During this time the patient may consume vast quantities of food, and certainly much more than would be eaten by a 'normal' person under similar circumstances. The preferred foods are high carbohydrate and fat preparations such as ice-cream and cake, but the bulimic is not limited to these. The eating is accompanied by a sense of being out of control, of being unable to stop eating or even to choose what foods are eaten.

One bulimia sufferer comes readily to mind. She came into the

Emergency room with an abdomen that *looked* painful. It was distended to the point of bursting. The skin was tightly stretched and shiny. She begged us to induce vomiting to relieve her obvious distress but we could not – we might have caused her to rupture her stomach. She told us how she got into this state. It started after dinner with a block of ice-cream, and was quickly followed by one large sliced pan, with butter and jam applied to each slice. She then ate two large cakes, another block of ice-cream, a few bars of chocolate, and a packet of biscuits. She forgot what else she had eaten. She had lost all control.

The patient with bulimia will do everything in her power to prevent weight gain. She will resort to induced vomiting, excessive exercise, laxative abuse or episodes of fasting. Patients with bulimia need expert psychiatric help.

It is also possible to suffer from binge eating without having full-blown bulimia nervosa. In these cases the binge eating may be exactly the same but it is not followed by attempts at weight loss. Warning signs that suggest you have a binge-eating disorder include eating rapidly, eating large amounts even when you are not hungry, eating alone because you are embarrassed about the amount you eat, and feelings of disgust and depression after a binge.

COMFORT EATING

Eating is always pleasurable. It satisfies a 'pleasure centre' in the brain. Indeed, the centre stimulated by the taste of nice food is the same centre that nicotine and cocaine stimulate when they are consumed! This suggests a very strong biological basis to craving. It is understandable that some of us would try to counteract unpleasant life circumstances by stimulating the pleasure centre with food. Unfortunately, it doesn't work. Researchers working with cravers and comfort eaters have found that they cannot improve their mood by eating (in the short term). However, if eating does not help them feel any happier, it must surely relieve some tension. It would appear, then, that comfort eating does not make us feel better; and yet we do it to stop ourselves from feeling worse. In the long term, comfort over-eating has a detrimental effect on body shape and size, and this subsequently affects morale and general health.

CARBOHYDRATE CRAVING

Carbohydrate craving is a feature of several clinical conditions including seasonal affective disorder (winter depression), bulimia nervosa, and the premenstrual syndrome. This observation led to the suggestion that individuals experiencing such conditions were subconsciously trying to increase the serotonin levels in their brains. The mechanism suggested for this effect was that high carbohydrate meals indirectly increased the levels of tryptophan in the blood; leading to more tryptophan conversion to serotonin, leading to a better mood. It was then suggested that some obese people who craved carbohydrate would fall into the same category, namely that they too were trying to self-medicate. However, it is not quite as simple as that. If patients with carbohydrate craving are indeed self-medicating with food, one would expect the positive mood effects to occur only in those who are depressed, and only then in the hours immediately after a high carbohydrate meal. But carbohydrate cravers are *not* able to improve their mood by single high carbohydrate meals. We also know that high carbohydrate diets given over three days have no effect on mood. However, several studies have reported beneficial effects on mood and energy from high-carbohydrate diets over 7–9 day periods. Conversely, diets high in protein may be associated with feelings of tension, depression and anger.

HUNGER AND THIRST

Craving for chocolate or other foods may get worse in some individuals if they allow themselves to get very hungry, for example if they skip a meal. Similarly, thirst is known to increase food intake during a meal, so drink a glass of water 20 or 30 minutes before you sit down to eat.

DIETS AND CRAVING

Contrary to popular opinion, dieting does not increase your cravings; it reduces them. There is an apparent contradiction here because we have just stated that hunger makes cravings worse! So how can dieting make them better? *Very* low calorie diets (in the region of 400 calories per day), and moderately low calorie diets (in the region of 1,000 calories per day) are both associated with reduced cravings *over a period of weeks*. As we all know, the first few days of any venture can be the hardest, so perhaps cravings do persist for a while. But as the diet progresses there is actually a reduction in hunger and craving. Patients with anorexia nervosa do not lie when they tell us they are not hungry.

BODY WEIGHT AND CRAVING

It is important to remember in all of this that the energy content of food never changes. It does not matter whether we eat it slowly or with undue haste, in tiny quantities or vast. Nor does it matter whether we eat under the compunction of normal hunger and appetite or abnormal craving. The energy content of food which we do not immediately need will be stored as fat. We might have been labouring under the burden of some of the conditions listed above, but they are not what made us fat. The eating is what made us fat. Fat is still energy stored, and it can be burned off.

Section 4

Health Effects of Diet and Exercise

14

The Benefits of a Healthy Diet

I t is well known that a nutritious diet is essential for optimal physical and mental health. Such a diet would contain adequate amounts of carbohydrate, protein and fat (macronutrients), as well as essential vitamins and minerals (micronutrients). Furthermore, the ideal diet would contain the correct balance of each of these various nutrients. Vitamins and minerals are essential for well being, not because they provide energy *per se*, but because they help the body to utilise the energy we get from macronutrients. They are also essential for the many biochemical processes that go on in our bodies all the time. Micronutrients cannot be manufactured in the human body, so it is essential that they are present in the diet.

From the point of view of being overweight or obese, we know that *how much food* we eat is important. This determines our energy balance. We want our energy intake to match our energy output. But from the point of view of our general health we know that *the kind of food* we eat is equally important. This determines our nutritional balance. For example, we can extract energy from the various carbohydrates, proteins and fats in our diet, whatever their source, and this energy will sustain life. But these macronutrients, and the foods that supply them, have other far-reaching effects on health quite apart from their role in energy provision. Let us take a closer look at the health implications of what we eat.

THE PRINCIPLES OF A HEALTHY DIET

A healthy diet is all about balance. Too much or too little of anything could lead to nutritional problems. There is now broad agreement on what constitutes a balanced diet. The key principles can be summarised under three headings:

- Major on the carbohydrates
- Go easy on the fats
- Eat plenty of fruit and vegetables.

Principle 1: Major on the carbohydrates

Carbohydrate foods should be the main constituent of a properly balanced diet. They should account for 70 per cent of total calories ingested. The main sources of dietary carbohydrate include:

- cereals, such as wheat, oats, rye, barley, maize and rice
- fruit and vegetables, all kinds
- milk and cheese, and their products
- purified carbohydrates, added to foods during manufacture.

We explored the biochemistry of carbohydrates in chapter 4. Briefly stated, carbohydrates include:

- the single sugar units (monosaccharides)
    - glucose
    - galactose
    - fructose
- the double sugar units (disaccharides)
    - sucrose (glucose and fructose)
    - lactose (glucose and galactose)
    - maltose (glucose and glucose).
- the multiple sugar units (polysaccharides)
    - starches
    - non-starch polysaccharides frequently referred to as 'dietary fibre'.

Glucose is by far the most important of all these sugars. The disaccharides and polysaccharides are broken up in the gut to release their single sugar units. Single units of glucose can be absorbed straight away; all other types of sugar are converted to glucose and then absorbed.

The best carbohydrates to eat are those with a low glycaemic index, i.e. those that cause a slow and gentle rise in blood sugar (such as potato, rice and wholemeal bread). High glycaemic foods are those that cause rapid and steep increases in blood sugar, such as sweets, chocolate, jams, etc.

Principle 2: Go easy on the fats

Dietary fats are an essential component of the diet: they are the most energy-dense food available, they carry fat-soluble vitamins, they are involved in cell membrane structure and function; and they are the basic building blocks of many important chemicals and hormones. However, because fats are so energy-dense (and taste so nice!) they are an important factor in the development of overweight and obesity. Furthermore, epidemiological studies show that fat consumption is correlated to death from stroke and heart disease. This effect is directly related to cholesterol levels: for every 0.026 mmol/l increase in cholesterol there is a 1–2 per cent increased risk of heart disease.

However, not all fats are the same, nor do they all have the same effect on cholesterol. Saturated fats are the most likely to cause problems because they have a clear cholesterol-raising effect. On the other hand, polyunsaturated fats (also called omega-3 and omega-6 essential fatty acids) and monounsaturated fats (omega-9) do not raise cholesterol levels. This is the reason behind the preference for using polyunsaturated as opposed to saturated fats. A simple rule of thumb is that saturated fats are solid at room temperature (e.g. butter) whereas unsaturated fats are liquid (e.g. olive oil).

For these reasons it is recommended that . . .

- fat consumption should be *reduced* from present levels to provide no more than 30 per cent of total calorie intake, and some experts would prefer reductions to 20–25 per cent
- no more than 10 per cent of calories should come from saturated fats
- the consumption of omega-3 fats (e.g. fish oil) should be *increased* from the present average consumption to provide 0.2 g per day (equivalent to one tin of sardines every five days).

Foods which contain fats include . . .

- oils, butter, margarine
- biscuits, pastry, cakes
- chocolate, sweets, crisps and savoury snacks.

Principle 3: Eat plenty of fruit and vegetables

A great deal of attention has been paid in recent years to the possible protective effect of certain foods, and particularly those that contain antioxidants. There is reason to believe that fruit and vegetables, which are high in antioxidants, can significantly reduce our risk of heart disease, stroke, cataracts and cancer. For example, there is consistent evidence of an association between *high* levels of heart disease and *low* levels of antioxidants, such as vitamin E, vitamin C and the flavanoids. This suggests that people with high intakes of fruit and vegetable (and hence high levels of antioxidants) are protected from heart disease. Similarly, there have been in excess of two hundred studies that strongly suggest an association between *high* vegetable and fruit intakes and a two- to four-fold *reduction* in the risk of many cancers. Apart from their protective effects, there are other benefits to increasing our consumption of fruit and vegetables: they are a convenient way of reducing our consumption of fats, and a good way to obtain more 'fibre'. All of this can be summed up in one simple piece of advice: we should all be eating at least four, and preferably five portions (400 g) of fruit and vegetables per day.

A WORD ABOUT PROTEIN

Although much has been written about protein in relation to physical strength and stamina, the fact is that we need very little protein. Just 0.75 g per kg body weight per day will meet most people's needs.

A WORD ABOUT FIBRE

Dietary fibre is good for us. It is recommended that we eat at least three servings per day. The foods which contain the highest fibre content are the wholegrain cereals, wheat, oats, rye, barley, maize and rice. The reason for such advice is the strong research evidence of significant health gains from the regular consumption of wholegrain cereals. Studies consistently show a reduced risk of ischaemic heart disease and cancer amongst those who regularly eat wholegrain foods, even if only one serving per day.

Highest consumers of wholegrain cereals have a 30–40 per cent reduced risk of heart disease compared to lowest consumers; and this is true for both men and women. One large-scale study further demonstrated a linear relationship between consumption and benefit: for every 10 gram increase in cereal fibre there was a 29 per cent decrease in the risk of heart disease. Furthermore, at least forty studies have been conducted on twenty different types of cancer in relation to diet. The evidence suggests that cereal consumption significantly reduces the risk of several types of cancer, particularly cancers of the stomach, colon, mouth, gall bladder and ovary.

Wholegrain cereals exert their positive effects on health by two mechanisms, namely local effects in the intestine, and distal effects on metabolism. For example, they . . .

- increase faecal bulk and reduce transit time
- bind carcinogens, ensuring they are not absorbed
- provide essential nutrients such as tocopherols (vitamin E) and selenium
- have a low glycaemic index, which protects against the metabolic syndrome
- help to reduce fat intake
- have a specific and measurable effect on cholesterol: just 3 oz of oats daily can reduce LDL cholesterol by 4.2 per cent.

In public health terms, eating wholegrain as part of a healthy diet could reduce the incidence of heart disease and cancer by some 30 per cent. These would be very substantial public health gains.

A WORD ABOUT ALCOHOL

Alcohol is a food. It provides 7 calories per gram. It is usually consumed as part of a drink which contains other foods, notably carbohydrates. Thus the energy content of an alcoholic drink can be substantial. Men in affluent societies derive an average of 6 per cent of their total daily energy requirement from alcohol. The figure for women is 3 per cent. On the face of it these figures may appear small. But remember that small daily excesses accumulate over the years and eventually amount to significant weight gain.

Modest amounts of alcohol may help to protect against heart disease. Larger amounts very quickly become detrimental to health. In extreme cases, alcoholics can obtain most of their energy requirement from alcohol but they do so at the expense of other nutrients and run into serious health issues from the toxic effects of the drug itself as well as the nutritional deficiencies associated with it.

The current recommendation is that men should not exceed 21 units of alcohol per week, and women should not exceed 14 units. One unit of alcohol is equivalent to a small glass of sherry, a standard glass of wine, a single shot of spirit, or a half pint of beer.

DIET, MOOD AND ENERGY

Several dietary factors exert a direct effect on mood and sense of well-being. For example, it has been shown time and again that deficiencies of certain nutrients can adversely affect brain function. Vitamin B1 (thiamine), vitamin B6 (pyridoxine), vitamin B12, folate, vitamin C, vitamin D3, selenium and iron all exert independent effects on mood. The usual effect of deficiency is to feel tired and depressed. Indeed, sometimes supplementation with these nutrients produces an improved mood, even in the absence of overt deficiency. For example, some women with premenstrual syndrome report significant therapeutic benefits from vitamin B6. Similarly, improved mood has been attributed to thiamine and selenium supplementation. Other studies have shown that (even clinical) depression is associated with essential fatty acid (omega-3) depletion, and that essential fatty acid supplements can improve the mood of depressed patients. However, too much fat in the diet can lead to sleepiness and fatigue.

The carbohydrate and protein content of our diet can also affect our mood and energy levels. For example, diets that are high in protein are associated with feelings of depression, tension and anger. Conversely, diets low in carbohydrate are associated with fatigue and depression, whereas high-carbohydrate diets are associated with improved energy and mood.

The enhanced energy and mood effects of a high carbohydrate diet require a *long-term* strategy. Single meals of carbohydrate do *not* lift the mood, nor do high carbohydrate diets eaten for less than seven days! We are fortunate, then, that long-term high-carbohydrate diets are not only good for us but they improve our general sense of well-being to boot.

THE CONCEPT OF A FOOD PYRAMID

All of the principles of a healthy diet described above have been conveniently incorporated and simplified in the concept of the food pyramid. If you follow the general guidelines of the pyramid you will be eating a balanced, nutritious and healthy diet. The basic idea is that foods on the bottom tier of the pyramid can and should be eaten often, whereas foods in the top tier should be eaten sparingly (see diagram).

The Food Pyramid

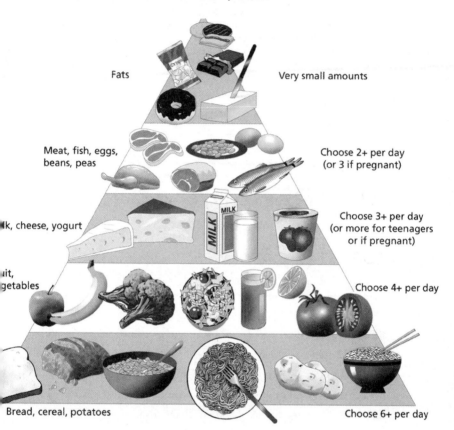

Fats — Very small amounts

Meat, fish, eggs, beans, peas — Choose 2+ per day (or 3 if pregnant)

Milk, cheese, yogurt — Choose 3+ per day (or more for teenagers or if pregnant)

Fruit, vegetables — Choose 4+ per day

Bread, cereal, potatoes — Choose 6+ per day

15

The Benefits of Exercise

Physical activity and exercise have enormous benefits for health. The physically active enjoy better health and longer lives than the sedentary. Notice that we are talking of actual physical activity, not just the concept of physical fitness. You may *feel* quite 'fit', and you may indeed be quite fit, but if you don't take advantage of your fitness by engaging in physical activity it will do you little good. Research shows that the *fit and active* are in better shape than the *fit but inactive*, although these are, admittedly, in better shape than the *unfit and inactive*.

This holds true even for the overweight and obese: it is much better to be overweight, fit and active than to be overweight and sedentary. Some studies have even suggested that it is better to be overweight, fit and active than to be lean and sedentary! In other words, you could be 'fat but fit and active'! And you could thereby enjoy better health and longer life than someone who is sedentary and lean. It stands to reason that the best of all possible scenarios is to be both lean and active.

So then, physical activity will have health benefits for everybody, regardless of body weight. And the activity does not have to be particularly intense or gruelling! Even 20–30 minutes of moderate physical activity three times a week will have an appreciable effect; although 30 minutes each day would be even better. By moderate activity we mean activities such as walking, gardening, cycling, housework, etc. It does not have to be any more demanding than that. Even so, very few of us are meeting the basic recommendations for physical activity. The World Health Organisation (WHO) has named physical inactivity as one of the most important risk factors threatening global health. WHO goes so far as to state that inactivity is possibly as dangerous to health as cigarette smoking! Three out of every four adults are at risk in this regard. At any one point in time, 75 per cent of people will confess that they have not engaged in any form of moderate physical activity for even one twenty-minute stretch in the previous week. This appears to be a well recognised problem because these same adults *know* that they are not getting enough exercise, and almost half of them think they should be taking *a lot* more exercise than they currently do. However, they still haven't done anything about their conviction!

What we are very good at, sadly, is watching television! Adults in affluent societies are watching an average of more than twenty hours of television each week. If we reduced our viewing by 20 minutes each day, and instead spent that time walking, we would revolutionise our public health data and our life expectancy!

People give different reasons for not partaking in physical activity. They cite pressures of time, finance, inclement weather and poor health, to name but a few. However, physical activity does not have to be formal and sporty, nor does it have to be continuous. We can increase our activity levels and improve our health by putting a little more thought into the everyday activities of life: walk or cycle instead of drive, get off the bus two stops before the destination stop, use the stairs rather than the lift, do a little gardening, walk after meals, watch less television, and so on.

The benefits of increasing our levels of physical activity are myriad and include:

- better sleep quantity and quality
- enhanced feelings of energy and well-being
- more effective stress and anxiety management
- prevention of further weight gain
- improved cardiovascular fitness
- improved lung function
- increased insulin sensitivity
- prevention (and improvement) of diabetes
- prevention (and improvement) of high blood pressure
- higher HDL ('good') cholesterol level
- lower LDL ('bad') cholesterol level
- reduced triglyceride levels
- faster clearance of fat from the blood stream after meals
- reduction in heart disease risk
- reduction in heart attack rates
- reduced risk of stroke
- reduced risk of several cancers, especially colon
- improved bone strength and reduced risk of osteoporosis (weight-bearing exercise)
- improved mobility and flexibility
- improved quality of life
- better life expectancy.

EXERCISE AND BODY WEIGHT

Physically active men and women are less likely to become overweight than their sedentary counterparts. This is partly because the active are more likely to burn as much as they eat whereas the inactive are more likely to burn less than they eat. However, the difference between the active and inactive extends beyond their expenditure of energy. The active are up and about doing things, burning off calories as they go. By and large, they do not eat during their activity. The inactive, on the other hand, are 'just sitting there doing nothing', at least in terms of physical demand, and they often eat during their inactivity! So they easily end up with a positive energy balance – a surplus which they store as fat.

The question we come to now is whether an increase in physical activity could help in the process of weight loss. From everything you have read so far in this book you would expect exercise to have a major influence on weight loss, and it does, but we need to qualify this. Moderate physical activities, such as walking, do not have a high energy demand. Another way of looking at this is to consider how efficient our bodies are at using energy. For example, you can walk at a cost of 360 calories per hour. But we must remember that the average adult male would have a resting energy requirement of 60–70 calories per hour anyway. So his net cost was only (360 − 70 =) 290 calories. However, if he didn't go for a walk he would probably have done something else, and he would have used up another 50 calories in the process. So now his walk has made a net difference of only (290 − 50 =) 240 calories. Furthermore, if he follows his walk with what he considers to be a well-deserved rest, and rewards himself with a snack, he would end up with no net loss of calories, and possibly even a surplus!

But we must not lose sight of this: he has gained all the benefits of the exercise. His heart and lungs will work better, his blood pressure will benefit, he will sleep better, and so forth. If he was careful not to over-compensate by resting and/or eating, and if he undertook this walk every single day, he would lose the best part of 10 kg weight in one year.

To depend on exercise alone as a means of losing substantial amounts of weight is impractical and may even be dangerous. The intensity and duration of the activity would have to be considerably increased beyond those required for a brisk walk. Such fitness levels are probably beyond the immediate reach of most overweight or obese individuals. However, if our subject was fit enough to do, say, thirty minutes on a rowing machine, then he could burn off 400 or 500 calories in one go. And if he was careful (a) not to overcompensate with prolonged rest after the exercise, and (b) not to reward himself with high-fat foods; and if he faithfully did this exercise every day, he would lose up to 450 g of fat in one week and up to 23 kg weight over the course of a full year.

Calorie restricted diets in overweight people produce much larger weight losses than can be achieved by exercise. As you might expect, the combination of diet and exercise produces more weight loss than either diet or exercise alone. There should therefore be equal emphasis on diet and exercise. Meanwhile, if there is only one thing you do for your health after reading this book let it be this: walk for 20 minutes three times a week. This simple measure will significantly improve your long-term health.

16

Diet, Exercise and Weight Loss

Most of us who are overweight or obese have gained weight little by little over the years through a combination of excess energy intake and/or inadequate energy expenditure. So what should we do now in order to lose weight? Should we 'go on a diet' (reduce our intake) or should we 'get out there and exercise' (increase our output)? The best answer is a little bit of both – there should be equal emphasis on diet and exercise in any weight-loss programme.

Rest assured, there is no need to go on anything that resembles a starvation diet, nor is there need to embark on a punishing exercise regime. In fact, each of these is fraught with danger. The best, albeit least popular, approach to diet, exercise and weight loss is patience. It took us years to accumulate our excess fat – we will not lose it all overnight. You may have become frustrated with your weight, and you may have suddenly decided that the time has come to do something about it. But notwithstanding the fact that sudden resolutions can be positive they have to be worked out and brought into reality over time. That will take patience. Your doctor, your partner, your employer or your children may have expressed impatience and put you under pressure to lose weight; but no amount of pressure will substitute for your own quiet and patient determination as you set out on a weight-loss programme. Besides, you're not doing it for them; you're doing it for yourself. You're doing it because you want to live life with more energy, more mobility, in better mood, with fewer health complaints and with a greater chance of seeing your grandchildren – and of being able to play with them!

The vast majority of rapid-weight-loss schemes are not successful. Sure, you might lose a few kilograms within a relatively short timeframe on some of these, but there is a 95 per cent chance that you will regain that weight within a few short years. Furthermore, you may even put on more than you lost!

WHY IS THERE SO MUCH FAILURE?

The main reason for failure to achieve and/or maintain successful weight loss is a failure to change the underlying lifestyle. Lifestyle got us into this state in the first place, and unless we change that we change nothing. We accept that genetics play an important role in all of this, but the fact remains that my physical inactivity, my television watching, my passive over-consumption of calories, my hectic lifestyle and my wrong choice of foods have caused my weight gain. This is not a popular message, but true nonetheless. I need to change my lifestyle, and I will not lose weight until I do.

THE PROBLEM WITH 'CRASH' DIETS

Diets for weight loss are designed, by definition, to put us into negative energy balance, i.e. they provide us with less energy than we need, thus causing our bodies to dip into fat stores and start depleting them. However, if the diet is severe and provides very few calories, our bodies are 'shocked' into a state of emergency. It is as if the body shuts down metabolic processes or at least slows them down dramatically. The net result is that our basal metabolic rate is significantly reduced. It has been estimated that a very low calorie diet of, say, less than 400 calories per day could reduce the metabolic rate by almost a third. Slightly more generous but still low calorie diets of less than 800 calories per day would slow metabolism by up to 20 per cent. Thus, very low calorie diets can be self-defeating: the less you eat the less you need! Besides, you can immediately see one mechanism for rapid weight gain when the diet is broken: the body becomes super-efficient at using and storing energy. This is one way in which 'dieting can make you fat'.

Another problem with severe diets is that much of the weight loss is from the non-fat parts of our body! On very low calorie diets up to 30 per cent of the weight lost will come from the breakdown of internal organs and muscles, with the remaining 70 per cent coming from fat stores. This explains the emaciated appearance of starvation victims, whether wilful or enforced. A more sensible diet, allowing 1,500 calories per day, would result in a 10 per cent loss from the lean body mass, with the remaining 90 per cent coming from fat stores. As you can see, some loss from lean body mass is inevitable even on a well structured and considered weight-loss regime.

Finally, the very rapid initial weight loss on these 'lose-weight-quickly schemes' is an illusion. It is due to fluid loss – it has nothing to do with fat, and everything to do with glycogen. Glycogen is stored in the liver and muscles, where each molecule of glycogen is attached to several molecules of water. Rapid utilisation of glycogen, such as occurs on a starvation regime, leads to the rapid release of water. This water is passed as urine and the body loses 'weight'. But that weight was lost from muscle and liver, not from fat stores.

THE PROBLEM WITH FAD DIETS

The main problem with fad diets, apart from the fact they are not scientifically-based, is that many of them are nutritionally incomplete. They are also difficult to incorporate into your everyday lifestyle. Bear in mind that whatever method you choose to help you lose weight will need to become part of your lifestyle at least for the foreseeable future.

THE PROBLEM WITH ALL DIETS

Eating is always pleasurable, no matter what the consequences; and fasting is always demanding. Nobody enjoys a diet. The very mention of the word evokes feelings of tedium and despair. The stress of dieting is even evident at a biological level: the stress hormone cortisol is elevated in people who are actively trying to lose weight. Calorie restricted diets are effective, but they demand thought and commitment. In the process, some people become obsessed with calorie-counting, and end up completely preoccupied with food. They spend the whole day thinking about what they are going to eat next, and when. This kind of calorie counting is a very unnatural approach to the hunger/satiety cycle. Besides, preoccupation with food is a sure path to failure: you simply cannot keep it up as a lifestyle; it will drive you mad. Moreover, low calorie diets may lower your serotonin levels, and your mood can suffer as a result. Thus, the low mood associated with dieting may be more than just the cranky effect of 'boring food'. Finally, many people attest to the fact that they overcompensate with reward foods when they eventually break their diet, and they end up putting all the weight back on again. This is the yo-yo effect, and it is very demoralising. The most successful diets are those which involve small but significant changes in lifestyle over prolonged periods of time. Eat less, exercise more.

Section 5

Methods for Weight Loss

17

The Medical Check-up

Our current health status and future health prospects, and even our life expectancy, all depend substantially on our body weight. Being overweight or obese are therefore extremely important issues. For this reason, it may be wise at the outset of any substantial weight-loss programme to enlist the help of an interested doctor. The initial medical assessment would provide you with

- an accurate assessment of your current degree of overweight or obesity
- a comprehensive assessment of your current health status, with particular reference to the complications of overweight and obesity
- the basis for a risk assessment of future health.

You will appreciate, given what we know about the potential health effects of overweight and obesity, that the initial medical assessment may take some time. This will involve a clinical history, a physical examination, and a few laboratory tests.

CLINICAL HISTORY

The clinical history will elicit any symptoms you may have in relation to overweight or obesity, and will also draw attention to any other problems that may be present. In particular, symptoms of diabetes should be actively sought as this condition is frequently overlooked. The symptoms include increased thirst, more frequent passing of urine, and fatigue. However, damage to vital structures occurs in diabetes even when symptoms are mild, so this should be checked for routinely. The symptoms of sleep apnoea and depression should also be sought as these conditions may be easily overlooked too.

An assessment of your levels of physical activity will give the doctor some idea of your current level of physical fitness as well as provide a base line for any future exercise prescription. It would also be helpful to discuss your reasons for wanting to lose weight. This will ensure that you are starting from a positive and realistic position, rather than from some burdensome sense of obligation.

The clinical history will include an assessment of other risk factors for heart disease and stroke:

■ Cigarette smoking
■ A family history of premature coronary heart disease (in males younger than 55 years, and females younger than 65 years at age of diagnosis)
■ Physical inactivity, defined as less than three 20 minute sessions per week of moderate exercise
■ Alcohol intakes above the recommended 21 units for men and 14 units for women.

PHYSICAL EXAMINATION

During the physical examination your doctor may wish to conduct the following:

- Height and weight measurements, from which your BMI is calculated
- Waist and hip measurements, from which an idea of central obesity is obtained
- Blood pressure recordings, including a 24-hour recording if appropriate
- Cardiovascular health assessment, including an ECG if appropriate
- Assessment for other signs of atherosclerosis such as
  - peripheral circulation disorders
  - abdominal vessel disorders
  - carotid vessel disorders
- Lung function assessment.

The doctor will also take note of the presence or absence of varicose veins, leg ulcers, varicose eczema, arthritis, urinary incontinence, etc. All of these could interfere in some way with the weight-loss programme and may need to be addressed in their own right.

LABORATORY TESTS

Laboratory investigations would include:

- Urine analysis
  - for the presence of sugar (testing for diabetes mellitus)
  - for the presence of protein (testing for kidney damage)
- Blood tests (ideally a fasting sample) for
  - Glucose

- Cholesterol
- Triglyceride

Tests for thyroid function and other medical causes of weight gain would only be carried out if symptoms or signs of other disorders were present. Otherwise there is simply no point in checking for these.

ASSESSING YOUR RISK

Clearly, the overall risk to your health is a direct function of

- the degree of your overweight or obesity
- the size of your waist
- your triglyceride and cholesterol levels
- the complications of overweight and obesity already present
- other risk factors identified, both genetic and lifestyle.

In medicine we talk of modifiable and non-modifiable risk factors. The good news is that most of the risk factors discussed in this chapter *are* modifiable. The only thing you cannot change is your genetic make-up. Everything else is subject to your control: you can stop smoking, you can increase your level of physical activity, and you can lose weight. If necessary, your high blood pressure and elevated triglyceride and cholesterol levels can also be treated.

ENROLLING IN A WEIGHT-LOSS PROGRAMME

Successful weight loss programmes are characterised by several features:

- They start from a position of care.
- They do not judge the overweight or obese.

■ They understand the complexities involved in the process of weight gain (and loss).

■ They encourage reasonable and realistic targets for weight loss, in the knowledge that even small losses have large health benefits.

■ They promote a change in lifestyle commensurate with the desired weight loss.

■ They place equal emphasis on diet and exercise.

■ They preach patience.

■ They encourage a network of friendship and support with like-minded individuals.

■ They provide frequent follow-up and assessment with an interested doctor or other health professional.

SETTING A REALISTIC TARGET

At this stage of the medical assessment you should have a clear idea of your current health status and your future health risks. From these you will know how much weight you would like to (or need to) lose, and you will have some sense of the urgency of that need. The fact that you may 'urgently need to lose weight' should never be a cause for panic. It just means that you need to *start* losing weight *now*. It does not mean that you have to lose it all instantly. Don't put it off. Sit down with your doctor, talk through the results of your assessment and discuss how best to approach the task. Some authorities recommend that you aim to lose 10 per cent of your current body weight within the first six months. Many people can achieve that rate of loss but some would find it difficult. Other experts suggest that a 5 per cent loss would be just as good in the first instance. The latter point out the greater likelihood of achieving a more modest goal; and that even small amounts of weight loss are beneficial to health.

A PRESCRIBED DIET

If appropriate, you will be offered a prescribed diet. Standard protocols are available, but a personalised diet administered by a dietician may be more suitable in certain cases. The idea behind any weight-loss diet is to restrict the number of calories in such a way as to make the body burn up its fat stores. Most prescribed diets restrict the total daily intake by between 500 and 1,500 calories. The calculations for weight loss diets are quite straight-forward, at least in theory. You can estimate your total daily energy requirement from your basal metabolic rate (BMR) and your physical activity level (PAL) as described in chapter 2; and you can then decide by how much to restrict your intake. We know that 450 g of fat contain 3,000 to 3,500 calories, so we can calculate a daily restriction in the knowledge that it will result in a certain rate of weight loss. Theoretically, eating 500 calories per day less than the total daily energy requirement would result in a weight loss of approximately 450 g per week. And that is a perfectly acceptable rate of weight loss: you would lose over 20 kg in one year.

A PRESCRIBED EXERCISE PROGRAMME

Most overweight-but-otherwise-healthy people can increase their activity levels without risk. The very inactive, the obese, and those with medical complications of any kind would benefit from an exercise programme designed specifically for them by their doctor. The most accurate exercise programmes are those based on 'target heart rates'. These in turn are calculated on an individual basis from your current body weight and age. In the initial stages of the programme you would aim to get your heart rate up to a certain minimal level, known as the 'lower target heart rate'. As time goes by, weight is lost, fitness is improved, and you can start aiming for a higher heart rate. These exercise programmes should be conducted under the direction of the attending physician.

REGULAR REVIEWS

Regular reviews with your doctor or other health professional will encourage you to stay on course and to reach your target. These visits will include an accurate measurement of weight loss. They will also give you an opportunity to discuss your progress, and the various practical and/or medical challenges that may arise along the way. Research shows that individuals who are actively engaged in a weight-loss programme with regular monthly reviews do best in the long run.

18

Getting Started, Getting Results

The first thing to do is set a target. This should be somewhere between 5 and 10 per cent of your starting body weight. Remember that a 5 per cent weight loss is easier to achieve; and even though it is less dramatic it will still have a significant health benefit. Besides, you can repeat a 5 per cent weight loss as often as you like until your desired weight is achieved.

Once you have decided how much you want to lose you can then decide how fast you would like to lose it. The fastest advisable rate of weight loss is 2 kg in each of the first two weeks, followed by a sustained loss of 1 kg per week thereafter. This suggests that the most anybody should lose in a six-month period is 28 kg, i.e. 2 kg in each of the first two weeks followed by 1 kg in each of the next 24 weeks. However, slower rates of weight loss are perfectly acceptable, so long as they are sustained. You will recall the potential 20 per cent difference in metabolic rate that can exist between one individual and another. This means that for each person who manages to lose weight at the fastest advisable rate, there will be another person, equally disciplined in relation to food and activity, who will lose weight at half that rate, i.e. 1 kg for each of the first two weeks followed by a sustained rate of 0.5 kg per week thereafter. That is still a perfectly acceptable rate of loss.

So, although you may start out with brave targets for weight loss, you may find that you fall into the slower rate of loss. If this is so, and you are being honest about your diet and exercise, then revise your targets. Don't blame yourself for what you cannot control. The graph below shows two women on a weight-loss programme. They had the same height (1.66 metres) and weight (85 kg) at the start of the programme. You can see that one of them is losing weight faster than the other. This is in spite of the fact that they are both eating the same type and amount of food, and both engaging in the same amount of physical activity. Their BMI was 30.8 to start with – they were borderline obese.

Variable rates of weight loss

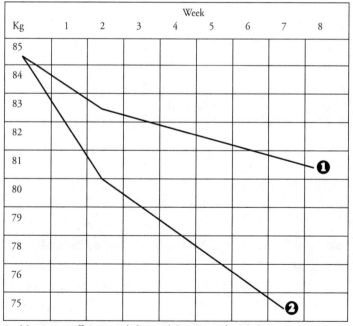

1   More energy-efficient metabolism and slower rate of weight loss
2   Less energy-efficient metabolism and faster rate of weight loss

SO, WHAT ARE MY OPTIONS?

There are several ways to approach the issue of weight loss. Choose the one which best suits your personal circumstances and targets.

Option 1: Diet and Exercise – lifestyle change

If you are overweight (with a BMI somewhere between 25 and 30) you could decide to simply and consciously reduce your intake of foods that are high in fats and sugars, and simply but consciously increase your levels of physical activity. If you do this you will lose weight. Of course, this will be true only as long as you do not increase your consumption of other foods. As far as weight is concerned, it is the total daily calorie intake that is important – not where those calories came from. Sugars and fats are high-calorie foods that are easy to identify and avoid; and they have little other nutritional value. They may be nice to eat, but we can easily get by without them.

Option 2: Diet and Exercise – medically prescribed

If you do not achieve your desired weight loss from following option 1, or if you are starting from a position of obesity (with a BMI greater than 30), and particularly if you have other health reasons for more urgent weight loss, you could opt for a more specific and comprehensive weight-loss programme. This would take your past and current medical history into account, and would provide you with a personalised prescribed diet and exercise regime.

Option 3: Diet and Exercise – an optional push-start

Having thus far paid homage to established doctrine in relation to weight loss and management, I would like to introduce just one gimmick. Please bear with me as I explain the rationale behind this little 'trick of the trade'. It is not offered as a validated scientific instrument, nor does it have any magical properties. But it is a very handy 'push-start' on the road to lifestyle change and weight management. Patience is important, but it's always nice to see some quick results as well!

THE FRESH FOODS DIET

The fresh foods diet, as the name suggests, consists only of foods that are fresh and in their original state. Thus, it allows all manner of

- fresh vegetables (including potato)
- fresh fruits
- fresh meats
- fresh poultry
- fresh fish
- fresh shellfish
- fresh herbs and spices
- olive and sunflower oils
- pure sea salt and ground peppercorn.

The recommended drinks are bottled spring water and herbal teas. Everything else is excluded: cereals, breads, dairy products, eggs, refined sugars, processed foods, etc.

This diet is most familiar to me as a 'detox' instrument in the investigation of patients with food intolerance. I have been impressed over the years with the number of patients who have lost substantial weight whilst using this diet in a bid to rid themselves of symptoms. This should come as no surprise as it is, after all, low in fats and refined sugars; and it easily lends itself to being a low calorie diet. But this is only true so long as the allowed foods are not eaten to excess (in order to compensate for the foods not being eaten).

As far as detox diets are concerned, this is quite an easy one to adhere to.

- It provides a great variety of taste and texture.
- There is plenty to eat so hunger is not a problem.
- It encourages large intakes of fruit and vegetables.
- The protein foods are filling.
- It encourages experimentation with fruits and vegetables that we may not normally eat (kumquats, mango, Chinese pear, dragon fruit, pineapple, avocado, salsify, asparagus, fennel, artichoke, etc).
- It takes us away from our over-dependence on high-sugar, high-fat foods.
- We begin to rediscover the taste of natural foods.
- We lose the symptoms of food intolerance (if we had them).
- We start to lose weight.
- We only stay on it for 4 weeks.

The Fresh Foods Diet has a few disadvantages. In the first place, there are two nutrients that are not fully provided for. These are calcium, which is an important nutrient for bone health; and fibre, which is important for bowel and general health. However, you only stay on the diet for four weeks. Thereafter the diet is expanded to include calcium- and fibre-containing foods. The second disadvantage is a practical one, namely that a lot of time can be spent in the kitchen preparing food. That's fine if you have the time; it's a problem if you don't. In spite of these drawbacks, this diet is a very good first step towards a healthy eating plan. It is also a handy way of losing up to 6 kg weight in one month.

Once four weeks have passed the diet is expanded to incorporate all of the principles of the food pyramid concept. Wholegrain cereals, beans and pulses, milk and milk products, and eggs may all be enjoyed at this stage. Where they exist, low-fat choices in these foods will help to maintain a steady rate of weight loss. Remember that all foods provide energy, so keep an eye on total calorie intake. Foods from the top tier of the pyramid are very energy-dense (high-fat, high-sugar foods) and should be avoided until you have achieved your target weight. Remember also that exercise is equally important as you follow this option.

GETTING RESULTS

Some readers will finish reading this book, embrace the lifestyle changes suggested herein, and lose weight almost without effort. Research in this area suggests that most adults will lose an average 11 kg over the course of the first six months of any well-structured diet and exercise regime. But others will struggle a little more with the process. Let us look at the possible outcomes (see graph).

1   You succeed, lose weight and achieve a normal BMI.
2   You succeed, lose a little weight but remain overweight.
3   You fail to lose weight but succeed in not gaining new weight.
4   You fail to lose weight and continue to gain weight, but at a slower rate.
5   You fail to lose weight and continue to gain weight, at the same rate.

Only the last of these possible outcomes could be considered an outright failure. The other four represent varying degrees of success. Those who succeed in reversing the process of weight gain to the point of weight loss have secured for themselves a substantial health benefit. Those who lose even more weight and achieve an acceptable BMI have secured the greatest benefits of all. But even those who succeed in preventing further weight gain have achieved a health benefit in so much as they avoid the accumulation of further health risks. The hapless individual who continues to gain weight misses out on the health benefits, and further increases his or her health risks.

So why do some people succeed and others fail? Because some enter a state of negative energy balance and others do not! The latter may

Possible outcomes of any attempt at weight loss

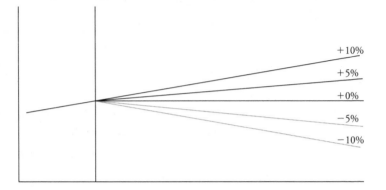

feel that they are depriving themselves of their favourite foods, but they are still somehow managing to take in as many calories as they are burning up. Everyone who is overweight knows how difficult it can be to lose weight. And some of them tell us that they simply cannot lose weight even when they stick rigidly to a diet. Let us immediately acknowledge that it is easier for some people to lose weight than for others. But we must also acknowledge that all who enter a state of negative energy balance will lose weight. They have to! So the confusion in these cases arises because people *think* they are on a negative energy balance diet when in fact they are not.

To investigate this further, some of these brave but 'can't-lose-weight' obese patients submitted themselves to research. They were invited to stay in a specialised metabolic unit as in-patients for several weeks. During their stay they ate only what they were given from the metabolic unit kitchen. Their calorie restriction was considerable, very accurately assessed on an individual basis, and consistent. They lost weight! Furthermore, when they went home to visit their families they invariably put a pound or two back on again! The results are paraphrased in the graph. Clearly, these individuals have difficulty losing weight because (i) they need relatively little to keep them going, and (ii) they have difficulty judging their food requirement and intake with accuracy.

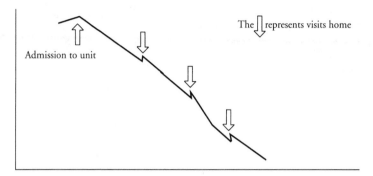

JUDGING PROGRESS

Whatever option you choose, you will want to keep track of your progress. The following charts give guidelines on acceptable rates of weight loss, with a particular view to preventing excessive loss. However, you should also be careful to maintain at least the minimum recommended rate of loss. Failure to do so suggests that the lifestyle changes you have chosen are insufficient to achieve your goals.

As you can see, the first month differs from the second and subsequent months in that it is characterised by a faster rate of loss. Once the body has made a few adjustments, a slower and more sustainable rate of loss will follow. If you wanted to, you could maintain this rate of loss until you reached your ideal BMI. Notice also that rates of weight loss may vary slightly from one week to the next. This is nothing to be concerned about. Failure to lose any weight in a given week is evidence that, for whatever reason, you did not achieve an overall negative energy balance during that time; and would prompt you to have another think about your strategy. If you are finding it all a little too difficult, and if there are good medical reasons for doing so, you should consider one of the medical treatments for weight loss.

Progress chart, first month

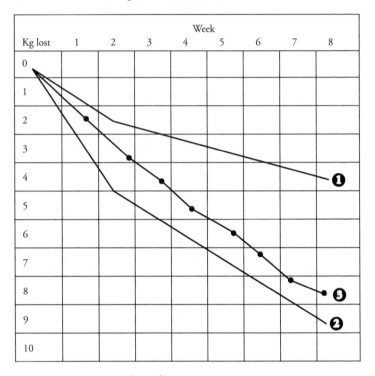

1   Minimum recommended rate of loss
2   Maximum recommended rate of loss
3   Example

Progress chart, second and subsequent months

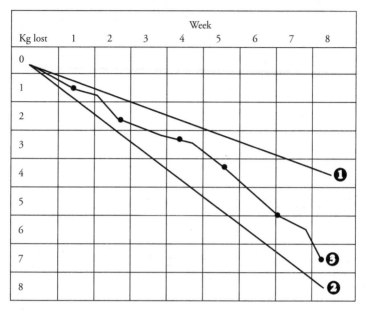

1 Minimum recommended rate of loss
2 Maximum recommended rate of loss
3 Example

Medical Treatments for Weight Loss

We usually think of 'medical treatments' in terms of curing or alleviating disease. We must be careful, therefore, not to lose sight of the fact that overweight and obesity are not diseases in the traditional sense of the term. If they were, we could hope for the discovery of a 'magic bullet' treatment that would rid us of our 'disease'. The fact that the global epidemic of obesity is a modern phenomenon is strong evidence that the root cause of obesity is a combination of genetic and lifestyle influences. For this reason, virtually all experts agree that the mainstay of 'treatment' for weight loss is attention to diet and exercise. Obesity is not a disease that can be cured with medicines.

However, although overweight and obesity are not diseases *per se*, they do give rise to many disease states, some of which are life-threatening. When these secondary diseases occur in the overweight, we do not hesitate to treat them. We will use medication or surgery, or both; and we would happily use any other reasonable means at our disposal to alleviate the problem. If we are so willing to treat the complications of obesity, why are we not equally prepared to treat the underlying cause of these complications, namely the obesity itself? There is a strong argument, therefore, in favour of treating obesity as if it were a disease before it gives rise to disease. This is especially important for those who are in the high risk categories, i.e. the very obese with large waist circumference and elevated triglycerides, or those with other risk factors such as personal or family history of heart disease, etc.

As things stand, it would be quite misleading to suggest that there is a simple medical solution to the problem. But there are some very useful aids. These can be considered under three headings, namely, medicines, surgical procedures and behavioural therapy.

MEDICINES

Early experience with medicines in the treatment of obesity was not satisfactory. They were mostly appetite suppressants, and although they had positive effects, they were also found to have potentially serious side effects. These earlier drugs, for the most part, have been abandoned.

At the present time there are only two medicines approved for the long-term treatment of overweight and obesity. These are sibutramine (Reductil) and orlistat (Xenical). Both are described as *adjuncts*, or aids, to the treatment of weight loss – *they are not a substitute for diet and exercise*. Research shows that these medicines can be a great help, at least in the short to medium term (6–12 or 24 months). That is, the addition of one of these medicines to a well structured weight-loss programme will secure more weight loss than diet and exercise alone. Each medicine has advantages and disadvantages, so your doctor will suggest the one that is most appropriate for you.

Option 4: Diet and Exercise and Sibutramine

This medicine comes in the form of a tablet which is taken once daily. All patients are given 10 mg per day during the first month, but this may be increased to 15 mg per day if the response is inadequate. This medicine is licensed for use in patients with a BMI greater than 30, or a BMI greater than 27 together with other risk factors. Unlike Xenical, it is licensed for use in patients who have not managed to lose weight by diet and exercise alone. Sibutramine works in the brain where it increases the levels of two neurotransmitters with the net effect of reduced appetite and food intake. Clinical trials have established that it works well and can produce a weight loss of between 5 and 10 per cent of body weight, depending on the dosage used, and on the kind of diet and exercise programme followed.

It also had other beneficial effects:

- reduced triglyceride levels
- elevated HDL (good) cholesterol
- increased insulin sensitivity.

Thus, sibutramine could be a useful medicine to help with weight loss in patients who have elevated triglycerides and diabetes (insulin resistance).

The side effects of sibutramine include loss of appetite, dry mouth, insomnia, weakness and constipation. Sibutramine also produces a small increase in blood pressure and pulse rate, so it should not be used in patients with heart disease or poorly controlled high blood pressure. Patients should be closely monitored throughout their treatment. Because it works on the brain, it should not be taken with other medicines that work on the brain, such as anti-depressants. Sibutramine should not be used for longer than one year.

Option 5: Diet and Exercise and Xenical

This medicine is taken three times a day, once with each meal. It works in the gut where it inhibits the enzyme (lipase) that digests dietary fat, resulting in an inability to absorb that fat. Thirty per cent of the fat content of each meal will pass straight through the bowel and be lost. The net result is a reduction in calorie absorption.

Clinical trials have shown that Xenical together with a slightly-low calorie diet (1,800 calories per day) can produce a weight loss of 5–10 per cent over six months, and an average of 16 per cent over the course of a year. The trials also show that much of this loss can be maintained over a two-year period.

However, there are fairly strict guidelines to its use. It is licensed for use in patients with a BMI greater than 30, or a BMI greater than 28 together with other risk factors. Even then, you must first lose 2.5 kg in one month by diet and exercise alone. This may appear somewhat fastidious but it does emphasise the fact that this treatment is an adjunct to weight loss, not a magic bullet. Once you have demonstrated some degree of lifestyle change, you are deemed fit to receive your first prescription for Xenical! Thereafter the guidelines state that a weight loss of 5 per cent should be reached by 12 weeks; and if this is not the case the medicine should be discontinued.

Adverse effects of Xenical are few because it is not absorbed into the blood stream. The most common side effect is oily spotting from the rectum, flatulence, fatty stools, increased defecation and, occasionally, faecal incontinence. These are usually mild and transient, and may be improved by reducing the fat content of the diet, and by using psyllium husk. Because of its inhibitory effect on fat absorption, fat soluble vitamins (A, D, E and K) may also fail to be absorbed and may need to be supplemented.

Xenical has other beneficial effects, including

- modest reductions in blood pressure
- reduced cholesterol blood levels
- reduced triglyceride blood levels
- better glucose control in diabetics and non-diabetics.

Xenical is very safe and may be taken for up to two years.

Option 6: Diet and Exercise and Surgery

Some patients continue to gain weight in spite of repeated efforts to lose it. They may become morbidly obese (BMI greater than 40) and are at ever-increasing risk of disease and premature death. Surgical intervention is an option for these patients and often their only chance of ever losing weight (and keeping it off). Only patients with morbid obesity who have failed to lose weight by all other means should be considered for surgery.

In the past, the only surgical treatments available for morbid obesity were very invasive procedures such as stomach stapling, gastric by-pass, and other major operations. These aimed to reduce the size of the stomach, or by-pass it altogether, and to reduce the absorptive surface of the intestine. Some of these procedures led to severe malabsorption problems, but may still be appropriate in certain circumstances today.

More recently, surgeons have been using a technique called gastric banding. This involves a 'keyhole' operation in which a silicone rubber band is placed around the upper end of the stomach to create an hour-glass restriction, and effectively reduce the size of the stomach that is available to receive food. This causes early upper gastric distension and, thus, early feelings of fullness. The net effect is reduced food intake.

The device contains an adjustable balloon, which allows the band to be tightened or loosened, without the need to operate each time. The intention is to leave the device in place permanently, but it can be surgically removed, if necessary. Although many patients experience side effects, the satisfaction rating is really very high, with 80 per cent declaring they were 'very pleased' or 'pleased' with the procedure and results. Approximately half the patients experience nausea or vomiting, a third complain of heartburn, and a few get abdominal pain. In some studies up to a fifth of all patients asked to have their band removed because of side effects.

Patients who tolerate the band lose, on average, a third of their excess weight, with some of them losing up to 75 per cent, over the first three years. These are good results. It should be noted that patients who are treated surgically still have to be careful with their diet and still have to engage in regular exercise.

Other devices have also been tried, with variable success. For example, some desperate patients had their jaw bones wired together to make it impossible for them to eat. But this did nothing for the hunger pangs; and I've met patients who got around the inconvenience by drinking milk shakes all day through a straw. They were wired, but they were still putting on weight.

Some surgical procedures for obesity are performed specifically to enhance one particular aspect of function. For instance, the surgical removal of a large apron of fat from a pendulous abdomen may improve the mobility of some patients. Liposuction is largely a cosmetic procedure and has no place in weight management.

BEHAVIOURAL THERAPY

All of the options for treatment advocated above involve some degree of common-sense 'behavioural therapy'. But lifestyles are difficult to change, even when we know that we should change them. Specific cognitive behavioural therapy, with a trained therapist, may be appropriate for those who want to change their most damaging habits but have not yet succeeded in this regard. It may be particularly helpful for those who tend to have erratic or binge eating patterns.

The majority of overweight and obese individuals would benefit from the simple camaraderie and support of a group of like-minded people who are taking positive steps to manage their body weight. For this reason, attendance at a local support group is often part of the most successful weight-loss programmes.

APPENDICES

APPENDIX 1: DIETARY INVESTIGATION FOR FOOD INTOLERANCE

The dietary investigation for food intolerance will take approximately 6 weeks to complete and will demand your full commitment and attention to detail throughout this time. It is therefore imperative that you choose six consecutive weeks from your diary which are free of important social occasions. If you do give in to forbidden culinary delights during the diet, you will undo all of your hard work! I would like to emphasise that this is the only reliable way to determine whether foods are causing your symptoms or not. It will be a sound investment of time and effort, and it may allow you to join the ranks of those who have found lasting relief from troublesome symptoms.

DIETARY INVESTIGATION FOR FOOD INTOLERANCE, STAGE 1

The first active step in dietary investigation is to rid the body of as many food allergens as possible. This 'wash-out' has two benefits. Firstly, symptoms that disappear may be considered intolerant in origin; and secondly, the body's reaction to the subsequent re-introduction of food allergens will be much more acute, thus enabling you to accurately identify culprit foods. Theoretically, the best wash-out of all is a total fast during which you drink only bottled or filtered water. This is a demanding task, however, and one which is not easily adhered to – especially by those who have domestic or employment duties. Fortunately, most patients do just as well by eating the Low Allergy Diet. This consists of ten foods, or so, which we know from clinical experience to be of low allergy potential, i.e. they are the least likely to cause allergic problems. Remember that commercially available foods may be contaminated with chemicals such as pesticides, herbicides, and fertilisers. These may cause symptoms in susceptible individuals. Organically grown produce is chemically free, and therefore ideal for the Low Allergy Diet. However, in practice most patients will do just as well on non-organic foods, but bear in mind that failure to obtain relief on this diet may be due to chemical sensitivity.

Withdrawal symptoms

Many patients who go on this diet experience withdrawal symptoms. A headache often starts on the evening of the first day, or during the course of the second day. On days 2, 3 and 4, muscular pains similar to those that accompany the 'flu are prominent (but not invariable). Fatigue and low mood are also common features of the withdrawal phase. You can avoid the unpleasant combination of caffeine *and* food withdrawal symptoms occurring together by slowly reducing your caffeine intake over two weeks *before* starting the diet. Needless to say, it is possible to contract another illness by pure coincidence whilst on the diet, so if you are worried about the severity of your presumed withdrawal symptoms, get them checked out by your doctor.

A word of caution follows for all patients with migraine, and for young boys with moderate or severe eczema:

Migraineurs: If you have ever lost your sight, or the power in a limb, or if you have ever had an epileptic fit during a migraine attack, you should *not* go on this diet without medical approval. The danger is that you would suffer the worst migraine attack of your life, and there is a small risk that this could leave you with permanent neurological damage. There are other options for you, and these you should discuss with your clinical allergist.

Boys with moderate or severe eczema: As mentioned above, one of the benefits of a wash-out phase is that subsequent reactions to food challenges are much more acute. For some unknown reason, young boys with moderate or severe eczema may become *exquisitely* sensitive to the allergens in cows' milk after a wash-out period. The imprudent re-introduction of cows' milk may then precipitate a life-threatening reaction. The correct procedure for a milk challenge in such cases is for the doctor to rub a drop of milk on to the child's lip, and wait for five minutes. If the lip does not swell the child is given 5 ml of milk to drink. If there is no reaction within twenty minutes, the child is given a greater amount of milk, and so forth.

A typical Low Allergy Diet starts off with the following (preferably fresh) foods:

- lamb, salmon, cod, plaice
- broccoli, parsnip, sweet potato ('yams'), turnip, courgette
- kiwi, pears
- olive oil for cooking.

■ bottled spring water only for drinking – natural (flat) or carbonated (fizzy).

The chances of inadvertently admitting culprit foods are reduced by further excluding all of the foods on this list that you eat regularly, that is, more than once per week. If, for example, you eat a lot of lamb, substitute this for duck; similarly, try runner bean instead of turnip, Chinese beansprout for parsnip, rice for sweet potato, well cooked cabbage for courgette, pineapple for pear, and melon for kiwi fruit. The fewer foods you eat, the greater your chance of success.

During stage 1, remember . . .

■ It may be preferable to conduct the diet under medical supervision.

■ Stay on the diet for 7–14 days, depending on your symptoms. Rheumatoid arthritics, for example, would need to stay on the diet for 14 days (and sometimes longer). They would also avoid meat.

■ If it's not on the list, you can't have it! As you see, no bread, no cake, no sauces, no cereals, no ice cream, no milk, etc.

■ You can eat any amount of allowed foods, in any combination, at any time.

■ You will be bored, but don't go hungry.

■ You need starch for energy – eat the sweet potato at least 3 times per day.

■ You should buy everything fresh. You can freeze it at home if you wish, because you won't add chemicals in the process.

■ Do not smoke. Do not drink tea or coffee.

■ If you use salt, it should be pure sea salt without added chemicals.

■ Use 1–2 teaspoons of Epsom salts for the first 2 days, especially if you are constipated, but not if you already have diarrhoea.

- Brush your teeth in bicarbonate of soda and water – toothpaste contains chemicals and corn. Put one teaspoon of bicarbonate into a glass of water, stir with your toothbrush and clean your teeth.

- Do not lick stamps or envelopes – the glue contains cornstarch and other foods.

- Check your medicines! Many drugs are packed in the factory with maize, potato, wheat, sugar, etc. Avoid them if you can, but do not stop taking a drug prescribed by your doctor without consulting first. It is dangerous to stop medication without advice.

- This is a diagnostic diet. It is therefore very important to stick *rigidly* to the allowed foods. This is *the only way* to find out if foods are causing your symptoms, or not.

- You may feel worse in the first few days with headache, muscle pain, fatigue and low mood. These are withdrawal symptoms. They feel like the 'flu. If they are severe, take soluble paracetamol and a hot drink of bicarbonate of soda (2 tsp in hot water).

- It would be wise to stay away from chemical exposures during this time. Remove all sources of chemical, namely, anything that smells – bleach, pot pourri, polish, perfumes, smelly soaps, etc.

DIETARY INVESTIGATION FOR FOOD INTOLERANCE, STAGE 2

The Low Allergy Diet will get rid of the symptoms of food intolerance! The very fact that symptoms disappear when you stop eating your regular foods is an indication that they were caused by those foods in the first place. Conversely, whatever symptoms you have left at the end of the Low Allergy Diet cannot be blamed on the foods you haven't been eating. Therefore, if symptoms persist, abandon the investigation and seek expert help. The possibilities are:

■ You are not suffering from food intolerance, and your symptoms are due to something else entirely.

■ You are very unlucky to be intolerant to something allowed on the stage 1 diet.

■ Your symptoms are compounded by chemical sensitivity or gut fermentation.[1]

You should only proceed to stage 2 if you have enjoyed a substantial reduction in symptoms! You are now in a position to test foods individually. The wash-out period of stage 1 accomplishes two things. Firstly, of course, it gets rid of your symptoms. Secondly, and just as important, it primes your system to react quickly to new foods as they are introduced. In other words, your intolerant reactions to food will be much more obvious now because your system has had a good wash-out. Any departure from this state of relief must be considered a reaction until proven otherwise.

In stage 2 (and stages 3 and 4), we will try to bring your symptoms back! We will re-introduce foods one by one, and we will identify your culprit foods in the process. Most reactions to the foods on the list below will occur within 5 hours of ingestion, although some foods, such as the meats, may take a little longer. Longer reacting foods are tested in the evenings. This gives them the evening, and the whole night to react (if they are going to react). Thus, if you wake in the morning with a symptom, blame the new food from the night before. The golden rules are as follows:

■ New foods should be tested *one at a time.*

■ Allow a 5-hour interval between each new food.

■ Eat any safe food with the new food, or in between new foods.

---

1 Described in *Could it be an Allergy?* and in *Feeling Tired All the Time.*

- Any symptom experienced during testing must be blamed on the last new food introduced.

- Watch out for headache, joint pains, wheeze, runny nose, itchy skin, depression, fatigue, diarrhoea, bloating, nausea, etc., and always blame the food – don't rationalise!

- If in doubt about a food, leave it out. It doesn't matter if a food is wrongly blamed because it can be easily retested (after a 5-day gap). It does matter if you unwittingly allow a culprit food to sneak back into your diet.

- If you get no reaction to a food consider it safe, and eat it as often as you like thereafter.

- If you do get a reaction stop testing new foods! And don't eat any more new foods until you are feeling well again. Continue to eat all of your safe foods whilst you wait for the reaction to subside.

- If the reaction is severe take soluble paracetamol and a hot drink of bicarbonate of soda (2 tsp in water).

- Re-introduce foods as follows:

Day	Breakfast	Lunch	Evening meal
1	Celery	Banana	Rice
2	Tomato	Carrots	Onion
3	Melon	Cauliflower	Beef
4	Tap water	Lettuce	Chicken
5	Oranges	Mushroom	Soybean[†]
6	Cow's milk, one glass	Cabbage	Turkey
7	Tea – one cup only	Apple	Yeast[¥]
8	Butter	Pineapple	Pork
9	Eggs	no new food[*]	Potato
10	Cheddar cheese	no new food[*]	Spinach

†   *Soak the beans for 8 hours, boil for 90 minutes, mash into minced beef and chopped onion (if safe) and make a burger.*
¥   *Crush three tablets of yeast into a safe food.*
*   *Eggs and cheese may take longer than 5 hours to react.*

Keep a detailed diary of foods eaten and symptoms experienced throughout the entire investigation:

New food tested	Time eaten	Symptoms, if any	List of safe foods
e.g. celery	*Monday 8 am*	*none*	*celery*
e.g. banana	*Monday 1 pm*	*headache after 30 minutes, lasted for 2 hours*	*–*
e.g. rice	*Monday 6 pm*	*none*	*rice*

DIETARY INVESTIGATION FOR FOOD INTOLERANCE, STAGE 3

We now move on to cereals and sugars. These are different from stage 2 foods, in that they do not always produce such an immediate reaction. They may take 2 or 3 days to produce symptoms. Thus, you could have wheat on Monday, Tuesday and Wednesday, and wake up on Thursday with a migraine. For this reason different rules apply, particularly in relation to the duration of each test. For the sake of variety, other foods are included here which will react within 8 hours of ingestion.

Day	New Food	Notes
1–3	Wheat	Test in the form of wholemeal pasta, pure shredded wheat, and/or homemade wholemeal bread [use wholemeal flour (no white flour added), bread soda, an egg (if safe) and buttermilk (if milk is safe)]. Some form of wheat must be eaten at each meal for the 3 full days.
4	Coffee	Use fresh ground, one cup only for breakfast.
	Pepper	Use black peppercorn ground on evening meal.
5	Cane sugar	Demerara or muscavado (the brown one!). Take 2 teaspoons at each meal for 1 full day.
6	Coconut	Use desiccated or creamed, with breakfast.
	Peanuts	Use the raw ground ('monkey') nut, with the evening meal.

7	Beet sugar	Use standard white table sugar. Take 2 teaspoons at each meal for 1 full day.
8–9	Corn	Use in two forms: corn on the cob and glucose powder. Also use homemade popcorn and pure corn flour if you like. Start each meal with fresh corn on the cob, and finish with 2 teaspoons of glucose powder.
10	Cauliflower	Eat for breakfast.
	Garlic	Use with the evening meal.
11–12	Oats	Test in the form of porridge, oatcakes and/or flapjacks (oat flake, safe sugar, butter). Eat some form of oats at each meal for 2 full days.
13	Malt	Use the extract, mix 2 teaspoons into a safe food at each meal for the full day.
14–15	Rye	Test in the form of ryvita crisp bread or pure rye bread. Eat some at each meal for 2 full days.

NB: Remember, if you wake up in the morning with symptoms blame the last new food from the day before. Abandon a test as soon as you are sure that a reaction has occurred.

DIETARY INVESTIGATION FOR FOOD INTOLERANCE, STAGE 4

You now know which staple foods are safe and which ones cause you trouble. We move on to stage 4. This is an open-ended stage, and it can go on as long as you like. During the first seven days we pay special attention to some of the chemicals added to food. Thereafter we test foods with multiple ingredients.

Day	New Food	Notes
1	White bread	(Test only if wheat is safe!) This is a test for anticaking agents, bleaching agents, etc.
2	Frozen peas	These are treated with sulphur dioxide and other chemicals.
3	Instant coffee	This is roasted over an ethylene gas flame and contains many chemicals.

4	Tinned carrots	If you are safe with fresh carrots, but react to tinned carrots in water (phenolic resin lining the can), you will have to be careful with all tinned foods.
5	Monosodium glutamate	This is used as a flavour enhancer, especially in Chinese food.
6	Saccharin	This is a sweetener hidden in some soft drinks and confectionary. Take 2 tablets as a test.
7	Raisins	These are treated with sulphur dioxide.

You can now proceed to foods with multiple ingredients. This includes jams, sauces, chocolate, cake, biscuits, etc. However, don't forget all of the other possibilities: cucumber, grapefruit, dates, asparagus, lemon, lentils, prawns, sprouts, chick pea, almonds, herring, sunflower seeds, etc. If you get a reaction from a food with multiple ingredients, you should be able to trace the source of your trouble (because you know your status with the main ingredients).

TROUBLESHOOTING

This is for patients who enjoy great relief from symptoms on the Low Allergy Diet, and then become confused during the re-introduction phase. Your symptoms may have recurred without clear-cut reactions. In the first place, let me say this: never lose sight of the fact that you have food intolerance! Get expert help if you cannot figure out your culprit foods. There are several sources of confusion:

1 *You have allowed a culprit food to sneak into your diet.* Go back to the point where you last felt well and eat only those foods that you are sure of. Stay there for a few days until symptoms clear again. Re-test the foods, but this time *take larger portions*.

2 *Your reactions take longer than 5 hours.* Go back to the point where you last felt well and eat only those foods that you are sure of. Stay there for a few days until symptoms clear again.

Re-test the foods, but this time *give them longer to react*. For example, allow one full day per stage 2 food; test wheat over one full week, etc.

3   *You have gut fermentation.* In this case symptoms will slowly return with a build-up of carbohydrate (starch and sugar) foods.

4   *You are drinking too much caffeine.* You had no reaction to one cup of tea (or coffee), you correctly thought you were not intolerant, and you started to drink too much of it. Stick to one cup of tea and one cup of coffee per day until the investigation is complete. Increase your consumption thereafter if you wish.

5   *Chemicals are accumulating.* Symptoms may result from the accumulation of natural and/or added chemicals as you expand your diet.

DIETARY INVESTIGATION COMPLETE! NOW WHAT?

You have now completed your dietary investigation for food intolerance. You have two options:

1   You can avoid your culprit foods. You may find that you can tolerate small amounts of your culprit foods after a prolonged period of abstinence, say 6–12 months. See what you can get away with!

2   You can opt for a course of enzyme potentiated desensitisation. This treatment will increase your tolerance to culprit foods, and if successful, will allow you to eat them without the penalty of illness. If you have had multiple reactions, or if your culprit foods are hard to avoid socially and nutritionally, you should give this treatment serious consideration.

Meanwhile . . .

■ Try to vary the diet as much as possible. This will help to prevent the development of new 'allergies'.

■ Regular vigorous exercise is beneficial to the body in general, and to the immune system in particular.

■ Beware of food cravings – they signal the emergence of new intolerance.

■ Pay attention to your nutritional status – you need adequate supplies of all essential nutrients.

APPENDIX 2: PROGRESS CHARTS

The first month

Actual body weight	Kilograms lost	Week 1	Week 2	Week 3	Week 4
	0				
	0.5				
	1				
	1.5				
	2				
	2.5				
	3				
	3.5				
	4				
	4.5				
	5				
	5.5				
	6				

For a personalised progress chart, please visit www.joefitzgibbon.ie

The second and subsequent months

Actual body weight	Kilograms lost	1	2	3	4	5	6	7	8
	0								
	1								
	2								
	3								
	4								
	5								
	6								
	7								
	8								

APPENDIX 3: A WORD ABOUT CHILDREN

The principles of energy balance, physical activity and a healthy diet are as important to children as they are to adults. However, infants and toddlers have special dietary needs and should not be calorie restricted, even if they appear 'fat'. It is reassuring to note that being very plump as an infant or toddler (up to the age of three years) is *not* associated with being overweight or obese in adult life. But we do need to be mindful of what happens thereafter.

The global joint epidemics of obesity and physical inactivity that are affecting adults are also affecting children. The incidence of obesity in childhood is increasing in most countries, and particularly throughout Europe and the Americas. Our children are going to grow up into an adult society beset by obesity, diabetes, heart disease and cancer. If we are going to make a difference for our children, we will have to tackle this problem of obesity *now*. Obese children are at greater risk of cardiovascular disease and premature death in adult life. Indeed, the early signs of cardiovascular disease can be found in up to 70 per cent of obese teenagers: they have higher blood pressure, higher levels of triglyceride and cholesterol, and higher levels of blood glucose than their lean classmates.

According to the World Health Organisation, many millions of cancers as well as cases of diabetes and heart disease could be prevented by encouraging our children to eat healthily, be physically active and stay slim. But physical inactivity is also a major problem in children. Almost half of all schoolchildren do not achieve the equivalent of 10 minutes brisk walking in any three consecutive weekdays – and the weekends are even worse than that! Teenage girls are at greatest risk. It is strongly recommended that all young people should partake in moderate physical activity for at least one hour every day. This is so important that many feel it should become a part of the routine day at school.

One great advantage in the management of overweight children is that they are still growing. This means that they do not have to lose weight as such, they simply have to grow into it. In other words, we encourage them to modify their lifestyle (increase their physical activity and decrease their calorie intake) whilst they continue to grow. As they become taller and stay at the same body weight their BMI will automatically revert to normal. We want to ensure no real loss of lean body mass, so no strict diets should be employed.

In terms of diet, all of the high-fat and high-sugar foods that promote weight gain in adults also promote weight gain in children. So does the number of hours spent watching television and playing computer games. Finally, if you as a parent are obese, your children are far more likely to be obese too. This effect is a combination of genetic and environmental influences. Perhaps, in view of the foregoing, you would consider a few lifestyle changes for the whole family? The health gains would be enormous.

Index